Breastfeeding
Facts
Over
Fiction

Health Implications on the African American Community

Mishawn Purnell~O'Neal, MPH

Library of Congress Control Number:2001117782
Purnell-O'Neal, Mishawn
ISBN 0-9712199-0-7
Includes bibliographical references and index

Table of Contents

Introduction

Many African American women have misconceptions surrounding breastfeeding. The lack of social and professional support continues to perpetuate many of the misconceptions. We find ourselves in the 21st century with adolescents, the parents of the future, never having seen an infant be breastfed or know of anyone in their family who has breastfed. As we look around hospitals, medical clinics and throughout our society, we are bombarded with images that promote the idea of bottle-feeding and the use of infant formula. To a much lesser degree, do we find information and endorsements surrounding breastfeeding. La Leche League, the organization that serves as the official group who advocates breastfeeding and its many benefits, does not have a presence in the African American community.

There are some that say that in a developed society such as the United States breastfeeding is not as important as in a developing country. They go on to say that the benefits received from breastfeeding are best felt in developing countries where infants have higher incidents of illness and disease, and are more likely to require medical attention. Unbeknown to many, a great number of African American infants who reside in developed countries live many of the same realities of infants who reside in developing countries and have just as poor health outcomes as infants living in developing countries. With its wealth and power the United States is no exception. The United States' African American infant mortality rate is 13.8 per 1000, compared to the white infant morality rate which is 6.0 per 1000 (National Center for Health Statistics, 1998). African American infants die at twice the rate of white infants before their first birthday. The African American infant mortality rate ranked the United States

1

at 40, below Poland, Bulgaria and Lithuania (Rosen, 1996). Developing countries such as Barbados and Jamaica, predominately black countries also have lower infant mortality rates than the United States' African American infant mortality rate (Warner, 1996).

This book shares with the reader information about the breast-bottle debate that is oftentimes not stated. The continued success of the African American community is dependent on the generations to come. The infant mortality rate and other health indicators lead us to believe that health outcomes for African American infants tend not to be as favorable as other ethnicities. From a public health standpoint, we must examine many of the factors that directly and indirectly impact the overall health of African American infants, which includes infant nutrition. I look to address the many misconceptions that surround breastfeeding from an African American perspective, as well as looking at the many historical factors that have influenced the attitudes and choices that African American mothers make when choosing how they will feed their infants.

This book also examines the infant formula industry and infant formula. The infant formula industry is a multi-billion dollar a year industry. The decisions that are made are made with the profit margin in mind and not always in the best interest of the infant consumers. We need to look at this question, and then answer, what would happen to the infant formula industry if all mothers decided to discontinue the use of infant formula and to begin to exclusively breastfeed? The answer is that the infant formula industry would be wiped out and billions of dollars would be lost. And because of this answer, it would stand to reason that the infant formula industry would work extremely hard to discourage as many mothers as possible not to breastfeed. As long as mothers rely on infant formula as they do, it continues the infant formula industries financial success. To sum it up, the infant formula industry has developed a product and they work extremely hard to maintain a market for that product. They are able to do this by deceptive marketing and advertising, by undermining the confidence of mothers and their ability to breastfed, and a host of other strategies to keep their product in demand. Unfortunately, the infant consumers of their products, which over half are African American infants, oftentimes cannot boast the same overall success from consuming their products as the financial success realized by the infant formula manufacturers.

Chapter 1

Misconceptions

Many of the misconceptions that surround breastfeeding have come from misinformation from health care professionals, family members, and from less than positive breastfeeding experiences that some women have had. Many health care professionals do not receive adequate training in the field of human lactation, therefore their knowledge regarding the physiology of breastfeeding is limited (Freed, Clark, Cefalo, Sorenson & James 1995). Their response to issues surrounding breastfeeding is to treat what they would consider to be a problem. A few of the common misconceptions:

I cannot produce enough milk
Human milk production is a complex physiological system. There are several milk production stages. Once in the lactation stage, there are two hormones that are necessary to produce milk, oxyotin and prolactin. Oxytocin is needed to stimulate the reflex of milk ejection, and prolactin is needed to stimulate continued milk production from the mammary alveoli. These two hormones along with nerve stimulants signals being sent to the hypothalamus in the brain by the suckling of the infant produces milk. It is very rare that you will find a mother who cannot produce milk (True insufficient, 1998; Hurley, 2000).

I cannot leave my infant if I choose to breastfeed.
There are many that believe that they cannot leave or be away from their infant, so they choose not to initiate breastfeeding at all. If an infant suckles just one times per day, it will maintain milk production (Hurley, 2000). Human milk supply is based on demand. Whatever the demand is, that is how much milk will be supplied. If that meant that the infant suckle times were peak in the mornings and in the evenings, the milk production and supply would peak at those times. With the many advances that have been made in technology, we have the capacity to express milk from the breast during times that the infant is unable to suckle. However, even for those who chose not to express milk, breastfeeding is still an option for infants based on the fact that milk production is maintained with one suckling experience per day.

Breastfeeding and Contaminants
There are those who believe that breastfeeding is unsafe because various contaminates can pass from the mother's milk on to the infant. This is true! Substances such as alcohol, tobacco, illegal drugs, environmental toxins, and over-the-counter drugs are passed to the infant through breastmilk (Hurley, 2000). There are those who say that this makes the mother's milk unsafe. Many of those same people who condemn breast milk fail to realize, or neglect to say that cow's milk, the primary ingredient of most infant formulas are subject to pesticides, hormones, substances placed in their feed and other possible contaminants. The most notable current addition to cow's milk is the genetically engineered bovine somatotropin (bST). The Food and Drug Administration (FDA), as a way to increase cow milk production, approved the bST hormone for use (FDA approves, 1994). The hormone is produced by a bacterium and injected into the cows. Currently the FDA does not require the labeling of milk that has been exposed to the bST hormone. Various organizations

have called for the halt of this practice based on the unknown risk. The FDA claims that there are no risk and continues supporting the use of bST. So yes, there are substances that do pass through the mother's milk and on to the infant. Fortunately, for the infant many of the potential substances that pass through the mother's milk, the mother has control over. None of the potential contaminant substances that are in cow's milk, and subsequently infant formula do consumers have any control over.

Breastfeeding and HIV Transmission

HIV transmission through breastfeeding is a current public health hot topic. There has been no consistency as it relates to the medical profession and/or advocacy groups as to the specifics regarding HIV transmission through breastfeeding. It has become pretty much unanimous that in developing countries where infectious diseases and malnutrition are primary causes of infant death it is recommended that breastfeeding be the feeding choice because of the low risk of HIV transmission compared to the risk of dying from other causes if not breastfed (Hormann, 1999). However, in developed or industrialized societies the statement is, women who are HIV positive should not breastfeed.

Much of the research attention has focused on HIV infected mothers and infants in developing societies and virtually no research have been conducted on the health outcomes of the HIV infected mother and infant in regards to breastfeeding in a developed society. There are many HIV infected mothers in developed countries, the United States included. The United States has the largest prevalence of HIV infected adults of any industrialized country (U.S Census Bureau, 2000). Almost 63% of all women reported with AIDS are African American, and African American children represent 65% of all reported pediatric AIDS cases (CDC, 2000).

It is the thought that in an industrialized society like the United States alternative feeding methods are readily available. The universal recommendation that HIV infected mothers in developed countries should not breastfeed is misleading and makes the assumption that all who live in an industrialized society have access and equal opportunities. This is not the case. Many HIV infected mothers in the United States are uninsured or underinsured, lack the financial resources to provide alternative feeding methods to their infants, lack safe and clean water in which to mix infant formula and overall have many of the same health related issues that face HIV infected mothers in developing societies. Current research has revealed that most infants are infected with HIV in utero or during childbirth, not through breastmilk (Breast feeding reduces, 1999). Infants who are exclusively breastfed do not seem to convey an excess risk of HIV transmission over formula feeding in the first three months of life, and mixed feeding carry the highest risk (Coutsoduis et al., 1999). It is thought that the introduction of solids may cause damage to the gastrointestinal tract of the infant which may create an environment for the virus to penetrate the gastrointestinal walls of the infant.

There are many HIV positive women who have breastfed and their children have not contracted the HIV virus. Researchers believe that human milk offers some form of protection from HIV infection transmission. The issue of the HIV positive mother breastfeeding should be explored. Although the health status of the mother must be taken into consideration, one example is when an infant has become infected at birth, breastfeeding may play a role in minimizing the occurrence and degree of severity of other infectious diseases seen in HIV-infected children, and in delaying the progression to AIDS in children who have acquired HIV perinatally (Black, 1996). This issue is significant within the African American community where there has been an increase in the number of women in their childbearing years that have become infected with HIV. The rate in which African American HIV infected women are giving birth is on the increase (Mofenson, 1999). Although there are drug therapies that are available to reduce the risk or perinatal transmission, a great deal of the therapy takes place during prenatal care, and this group is least likely to seek prenatal care.

Researchers, the medical profession and advocacy groups must take a closer look at breastfeeding for the HIV infected mother and infant in a developed society. The infants who are born to the HIV infected mothers, whether they are HIV positive or not should be provided with options regarding breastfeeding and the use of human milk. One option is the pasteurization or heating of breast milk. Heating expressed breast milk to 62.5 degreed C for 30 minutes or brief boiling the milk, followed by cooling kills the HIV virus, but retains most of the nutrients and vitamins (Hormonn, 1999). With the exception of the expressing the milk, heating of the milk does not require any more additional effort than the preparation that would be needed to mix and prepare infant formula. The use of banked human milk is another option. The many benefits that human milk offers would seem to be crucial to infants facing various potential health complications: greater susceptibility to infections, central nervous system damage, language, cognitive and motor development delays and a host of other issues.

Breastfeeding and Nutritional Status
The nutritional status of African American women and their ability to produce quality milk for their infants have been in question for centuries. As research has evolved it has shown over and over that the nutritional status of the mother is not the primary indicator of her ability to produce milk (Hurley, 2000). This is evident when we look

at the famine seen in various African countries. Generations have survived on breastfeeding even when the mother's nutritional status had been extremely low or marginal. Research has been conducted which showed that many of the protective properties of human milk are at very high levels even though the mother's nutritional status was marginal (Hennart, Brasseur, Delogne-Desnoeck, Dramaix & Robin, 1991).

I don't' know if a breastfed child has had enough to eat.

Another misconception that seems to make mothers want to bottle-feed as apposed to breastfeeding is the thought that they don't know if the infant has had enough to eat. Breastfed infants control the quantity of the milk that they receive, compared to bottle-fed infants whose feedings and intake are controlled by others. The tendency for the breastfed infant to be overfed is highly unlikely. Oftentimes individuals equate an empty bottle with the infant having had enough to eat and having a "good sleep" and they will continue to encourage the infant to eat until the contents of the bottle is gone. Maternal control over feeding is associated with an increase in adipose tissue which could possibly pre-dispose the infant for obesity later in life (Fisher, Smiciklas-Wright, Picciand, Frances, 2000).

Breastfed infants are too attached

Another widespread misconception about breastfed infants is that breastfeeding causes infants to become spoiled and too attached to their mother. Although to some this may seem like a bizarre misconception because when looking at many species of animals, the newborn more than not are very attached to their mother. Infants of the mammalian species have specific patterns that they use in an effort to maintain contact with their mother. Nursing infants tend to be responsive to the breast odors produced by lactating women. The olfactory system of various species is considered to be very

9

important. The sense of smell for many animals could mean life or death. For human infants, there has been less emphasis placed on the role of the olfactory system as it relates to their behavior. Recently there has been a great deal of research that supports the premise that through the sense of smell breastfed infants, especially in their first days of life, are able to recognize the smell of their mother and through their behavior able to demonstrate a preference for their mother (Fleming, 1998). This recognition of the mother is thought to be the initial stage of the mother-infant attachment process. Research has also documented that three-day old infants prefer to look at the face of their own mother to that of another mother (Blass, 1994). Another component of the mother infant bond that is facilitated in breastfeeding is the close skin contact. The close skin contact that is shared during breastfeeding favors a more gradual transition from the uterus to the extrauterine environment, because the infant is familiar with the mother's temperature and heart sounds (Uauy & Andraca, 1995).

The maternal behavioral response that breastfed infants exhibit involves complex, biochemical mechanisms. To associate the interaction between the mother and breastfed infant as one of over-attachment and being spoiled, would be disregarding the complexity of the mother-infant bond. Unfortunately, since breastfeeding is not the norm in our society, the behaviors that breastfed infants exhibit are all too often mischaracterized. Most infants in our society are bottle-fed and receive infant formula as their primary nutrition and the many behavioral norms that are considered acceptable are based on the behaviors of formula-fed infants. When in actuality the behaviors that are exhibited by the breastfed infants are natural responses and are derived from neurochemical sensory within their body.

Breastfeeding is only beneficial for newborns and in early infancy.

There are many who believe that breastfeeding is only important or beneficial in the first months of life. Infants receive many benefits from breastmilk throughout their infancy and as they transition from an all milk diet to one that includes solid foods. This transition period is extremely important because infants are at increased risk of developing various deficiencies, and not receiving adequate energy/caloric intakes from their diet. Many people believe that breastmilk can be replaced by cow's milk to meet the dietary needs of older infants. There are several potential health related problems with older infants consuming cow's milk. Cow's milk is a poor source of iron and could increase the risk of the infant developing iron deficiency or iron deficiency anemia. The use of whole cow's milk in the second half of life is associated with intestinal blood loss in a large number of normal infants and the amount of iron that is lost is significant (Udall & Suskind, 1999). Cow's milk is also associated with being a potential trigger for Type I diabetes in infants who are carriers of the gene (Marincic, McCune, Williams, Hendricks, 2000).

Another issue associated with the early weaning of breastfeeding is the potential for inadequate digestion and absorption of the foods from an adult diet. Adult humans have 32 teeth, all which have a specific role in breaking down food. When adults have teeth that are missing or decayed, there is the possibility that the food they have eaten will not be adequately broken down, digested and absorbed. If the food that is eaten is not absorbed, then the body cannot benefit from the nutrients that the food provides. This holds true for infants as well. Most infants at 12 months of age do not have the teeth necessary to adequately break down solid foods. Therefore the amount of food that is actually absorbed is less than that consumed.

This would place infants at great risk of deficiencies at a time when their bodies are going through rapid growth and development. However the infant that is still receiving breastmilk during this transition period is still receiving a food that is; easily digested and absorbed, contains the appropriate levels of vitamins and minerals, provides the necessary fatty acids and provides the older infant with an adequate energy intake when combined with other foods. A research study showed that 22% of 12 month olds and 33% of 18 month olds were consuming diets providing less than 30% of their energy coming from fat (Picciano et al., 2000). This is important because of the association between infant fat intake and growth. Breastfeeding should be considered the bridge that infants use to make a healthy transition from an all milk-diet to one that includes adult foods

African Americans infants should not be breastfed because they are at risk of developing rickets.
There have been widespread reports about the resurgence of rickets. Rickets is a calcium deficiency caused by a deficiency in Vitamin D. Much of the information that has been reported to the public about Vitamin D and breastfeeding has failed to give a full account of Vitamin D. Many of the reports have stated that African American infants that are breastfed are at increased risk of developing rickets. Vitamin D is considered to be a vitamin and a hormone. It is considered a hormone because the body is able to synthesize vitamin D with adequate expose to ultraviolet rays from the sun. Breastfed African American infants, particularly those who have darker skin, and do not receive adequate exposure to the sun are at increased risk of developing rickets (McCaffree, 2001). Even with that information, breastfeeding is the best nutritional choice for African American infants. As the campaigns continue to encourage African American mothers to breastfed and as the breastfeeding rates increase, health

12

care professionals need to make sure that they are explaining the need for infants to receive adequate exposure to the sun. Many health care professionals are not discussing this issue with African American mothers. The first line of defense is to recommend that all breastfed infants, especially African American infants, be given Vitamin D supplements (Tucker, 2000). With thirty minutes of exposure to the sun, supplementation is not needed (Smolin & Grosvenor, 2000). The news media continues to report that breastfed African American infants are developing rickets. Many of these reports are failing to link the development of rickets to environmental causes: limited exposure to sunlight, use of sunscreen, clothing covering the body, the season and tall buildings blocking the sun. Breastfeeding and breast milk is not the problem! This is just another issue that is being used to undermine the confidence of African American mothers and the adequacy of breastfeeding within the African American community. It is interesting and ironic that we never hear of reports about the potential risk of infant formula for African American infants.

Preterm or Low-Birth Weight Infants cannot/should not be breastfed

Many people, medical professionals included, do not advocate that preterm or low-birth weight infants should be breastfed. This is an issue that must be addressed especially because of the significant impact that it has on the African American community. Preterm delivery (before 37 weeks gestation) and low-birth weight (less than 5.5 lbs) remains the most important cause of neonatal death in the United States, particularly among African Americans (Beck-Sague, Morse, Stephen, 1996). African American infants are 1.8 times more likely to be born preterm than white infants (Low birth weight, 1999). The long-term health outcomes for preterm and low-birth weight infants include neurodevelopment deficits, learning disabilities, behavior problems and lower respiratory tract infections (Beck-Sague et al., 1996).

There is a great deal of history that surrounds infant nutrition and the pre-term and low-birth weight infant. In the late 19th and early 20th century, a premature infant that was not breastfed would surely die. This problem was so prevalent that wet nurses and human milk banks were established to provide human milk for these infants. Dr. Hess began the first center for premature infants in the United States out of Michael Reese Hospital in Chicago, and in 1922 he published the first book on premature infants. He made recommendations regarding infant feedings for preterm and low-birth weight infants and clearly human milk was the recommended choice of feeding for these infants. In 1940 a researcher concluded that premature infants fed a diluted half-skimmed cow's milk formula gained more weight more rapidly than those fed human milk (Greer, 2001). The premise was that the higher protein content in cow's milk increased the growth rate. Another researcher stated that unsupplemented human milk was not the preferred feeding choice for premature infants because it did not support the growth of their skeleton. As a result in 1958, Dr. Hess in his revision of his second book, chose not to focus as much attention on the use of human milk but to expand the focus on the use of artificial milk. In the early 1970s there was research that supported the fact that preterm infants fed human milk grew as well as those infants who had received formula. It was also questioned as to whether or not the ideal weight of gain for the preterm infant outside of the uterus was the weight gain that would have been gained had the infant been delivered at full term (Greer, 2001). Despite this questioning, the American Academy of Pediatrics (AAP) in 1977, came out with its first statement on the nutritional needs of the low-birth weight infant " the optimal diet for the low-birth weight infant may be defined as one that supports a rate of growth approximating that of the third trimester of intrauterine life, without imposing stress on the developing metabolic or excretory systems AAP, 1977 (Greer, 2001). This statement by the AAP set the stage for the almost exclusive use of infant formula over that of human milk for the preterm or low-birth weight infant

The classification of preterm oftentimes lumps all infants born before 37 weeks gestation into one category. Most preterm infants born at 35 weeks gestation can be breastfed. Those infants born between 32 and 35 weeks gestation can almost always be successfully breastfed, or at least given breast milk by bottle or tube feeding if necessary (The low-birth, 1990). Unfortunately for preterm infants, as a standard practice most are routinely fed preterm infant formula regardless of their gestational age. Infants that are exclusively fed preterm formula undoubtly grow more quickly, but there seems to be a misconception among many that this growth translates into a neurological advantage (Williams, 1993). Since the early 1980s it has been clearly established that low-birth weight infants fed their own mother's milk had an improved growth rate over that of donor human milk (Gross, 1983). Maternal milk of mothers who have delivered preterm infants has a very different composition of milk when compared to the maternal milk of a mother who has delivered a term infant. Preterm human milk provides substantially higher levels of various components which would provide enough energy, protein, sodium, chloride, and potassium to support growth rates in preterm infants approximating those of the third trimester of intrauterine life (Gross, 1983). This is extremely important for the future growth, developed and overall health outcomes for the low-birth weight infant. The preterm infant is at risk for many health complications that human milk can play a significant role in reducing:

- *Immunological Protection*

The low-birth weight infant is at great risk of developing various illnesses and health complications. The immunological components of human milk are essential ingredients that can aid the infant in defending off potential invaders of its body.

- *Neurological Development*

Several researchers have shown that there is a neurological development difference in preterm infants fed their own mothers milk over preterm infants fed formula. Preterm infants fed their own mothers milk has been shown to have an IQ advantage of 8.3 points over preterm infants fed preterm formula at 7.5-8 years of age (Williams, 1993).

- *Docoshexanoic (DHA) Deficiency*

The transfer of DHA, a long chain fatty acid that is essential to visual and brain development, takes place during the last trimester of pregnancy. Infants born premature are at risk of DHA deficiency, which could result in poorer vision and compromised brain and neurological development. Human milk is a natural source of DHA, and it is not currently found in infant formula in the United States.

- *Iron Deficiency*

Premature infants are at increased risk of developing iron deficiency, because they are all to often born before they can build up adequate iron stores. Preterm infants oftentimes only have iron stores enough for 2 months (Raji, Eyler, & Goenflo, 1998). The iron from human milk is highly absorbed in comparison to infant formula, which would decrease the risk of the preterm infant developing iron deficiency or iron deficiency anemia.

- *Sudden Infant Death Syndrome (SIDS)*

Infants born before term who are low-birth weight are at increased risk for SIDS, and the risk increases with decreasing gestational age or birth weight (American Academy, 2000). Breastfeeding has been shown to have a protective affect against SIDS (Ford et al., 1993).

- *Necrotizing Enterocolitis*

Necrotizing Entercolitis is the most common serious gastrointestinal disease seen in neonatal intensive care units, with a reported death rate of 20-40% (Lucas, 1990). Preterm or low-birth weight is the most consistent reported associated factors surrounding the disease (Lucas, 1990). It is suggested that human milk may offer the breastfed infant a degree of protection from the disease. The gastrointestinal tract (GI) of an infant is functionally immature, not fully closed, and without immune protect at birth (Wagner, 1996). It may take several weeks for the GI to close, and this is especially important for preterm infants. Whether or not an infant is breastfed or formula-fed may play a role in how the GI actually matures and the development of the infant's own immune system. The maturation process of the GI appears to be greatly influenced by the various bioactive substances and live cells in human milk (Wagner, 1996). Infants who are only fed infant formula are 6-10 times more likely to develop necrotizing entercolitis than infants fed only breast milk (Lucas, 1990).

- *Sepsis*

Neonatal sepsis is a very serious bacterial infection within the blood. Almost half of the sepsis-associated deaths occur to preterm infants. Because of the higher rate of prematurely within the African

American community, African American infants are 2.5 times more likely to die with sepsis than white infants, with African American males having the highest death rates (Stroll, Homan & Schuchart, 1998). Human milk has been shown to have a protective effect against sepsis in preterm and full-term infants (El-Mohandes, Picard, Simmens & Keiser, 1997; Wright, 1998).

For the last several decades, preterm infant formula has been the primary nutrition for preterm infants. The 1980s and 1990s saw the development of commercial human milk fortifiers for preterm infants. Human milk fortifiers are supplementations that are added to human milk. The theory behind human milk fortifiers is that by adding supplemental protein, vitamins and minerals to human milk, the preterm infant would be able to meet the third trimester intrauterine growth rate. Many hospitals are stocking their maternity units with human milk fortifiers and this is becoming the preferred feeding choice for many physicians. However, just as infant formula had and has many developmental problems, human milk fortifiers also have many biological issues that may pose the preterm infant problems:

- Human milk varies greatly from mother to mother. Adding supplementation to human milk may place some infants with upper levels of protein and/or vitamins and mineral and might place some others with inadequate levels.

- Supplementation of human milk may also compromise the biological components and antibody mechanisms that are present in human milk.

- Supplementation of human milk may also affect the GI and its tolerance for human milk.

- The current supplementation level of minerals in human milk fortifiers in the United States is considered to be very high. It is almost double the levels of some European countries. This higher mineral content is thought to lower the absorption of fat in infants fed human milk fortifiers (Schanler, Shulman & Lau, 1999).

There are many unresolved issues surrounding the use of human milk fortifiers. It has not been clearly established as to which preterm infants should be fed human milk fortifiers. In much of the research surrounding human milk fortifiers, the authors oftentimes speak of low-birth weigh infants and very low birth weight infants (less than 3.5lbs) as if they are within the same group, with the same feeding needs. There also needs to be much more research in the area of human milk fortifiers. Above all, even more emphasis needs to be placed on the delivery of information regarding the benefits of human milk for preterm infants, and to support and encourage mothers with preterm infants to breastfed or to offer their preterm infant their own breast milk.

Currently there are no nutritional requirements for the growth needs of premature infants that have been established that are comparable to that of breastfed term infants. However throughout the last decade it has been noted that the preterm/low-birth weight infant may have more at stake through various illnesses and other complications, and the concentration on the growth rate being comparable to the intrauterine rate may not be the tool that should be used to determine the infant nutrition that is suitable for the preterm/low-birth weight infant. The AAP addressed this issue in its 1998 statement "initially after birth, the management of acute neonatal illnesses and gradual advancement of feeding to minimize the risk of feeding-related complications such as necrotizing enterocolitis, many conflict with the nutritional goals of obtaining rapid growth in preterm infants" (Greer, 2001).

Too many preterm infants are not exposed to the benefits of human milk. Many hospital and physicians rely solely on premature infant formula and now human milk fortifiers. There are health complications that inhibit some preterm infants from being breastfed. However, there are a great many of these infants that can be breastfed or provided preterm human milk, that are not! Breastfeeding can have a definite role in the lives of the preterm/low-birth weight infant. The use of human milk for these infants has many advantages. In addition to the benefits received from human milk that are specific to the needs of the preterm/low-birth weight infant, there are many other benefits short and long term that's received by the term infant that is realized for these infants as well. With the preterm rate being significantly higher within the African American community, it is imperative that mothers, health care professionals and others recognize how important human milk is to the lives of preterm infants.

Breastfed infants do not grow as well as formula-fed infants
Breastfed and formula-fed infants tend to grow at similar rates in the first 3-4 months of life (Lo, 1996). In the months to follow, breastfed infants tend to grow slower and formula-fed infants tend be heavier. Within the African American community, it has been culturally accepted to view a larger infant as a healthier infant. When a breastfed infant is compared in weight with a formula-fed infant it seems as if the breastfed infant is not growing and the formula-fed

infant is. Infant formula is made from cow's milk which has a higher protein level. This level is high enough to support the doubling of the weight of a calf in approximately 2 months. Human infants do not double their weight until the 4th or 5th month, and as a result the protein level in human milk is quite lower than that found in cow's milk and infant formula. In actuality it is not that the formula-fed infant is healthier because it is heavier, but that the breastfed infant is actually growing based on the natural growth rate for the human species.

Breastfeeding increases the risk of developing Jaundice
There are many who believe that breastfeeding is a contributing factor to the development of neonatal jaundice. There has been an increase in the number of newborn breastfed infants who have been readmitted to hospitals after discharge with the diagnosis of jaundice. Excessive plasma levels of red blood cells cause jaundice. These elevated levels produce a yellow-orange pigment called bilirubin. In some infants the liver is unable to break down the levels of bilirubin and as a result there is a development of jaundice that causes the skin and the eyes to take on a yellowish-orange color. In adults the normal level of bilirubin is 1 mg per deciliter, and newborns are considered to be jaundice if they have levels higher than 5-6mg per deciliter (Gillis, 1993). Nearly every infant born develops elevated levels of bilirubin in the first two weeks of life, which is called physiologic jaundice. In the first two weeks of life there is no statistical difference in levels of jaundice between formula-fed infants and those who are breastfed effectively (Hertz, 1999).

Breastfeeding jaundice is the name given to the exaggeration of physiologic jaundice that occurs in breastfed infants when there is an inadequate intake of milk and calories (Gartner & Lee, 1999). Breastfeeding jaundice that occurs within the first weeks of life is associated with the infant not receiving enough milk and calories which leads to weight loss and an increase in the bilirubin levels. Unfortunately, because many physicians and health professional do not have a clear understanding of breastfeeding techniques and management they are unable to offer support to the breastfeeding mother. As a result this may lead to ineffective breastfeeding management; infant not suckling enough times per day, infant being given supplemental food and/or water, infant not latched on properly to receive milk and many other breastfeeding management issues. The misconception around breastfeeding and jaundice is that oftentimes when breastfed infants who have elevated levels of bilirubin are taken off the breast and given infant formula there is a decline in the bilirubin levels. Weight loss is associated with increased bilirubin levels, which is usually seen in the breastfed infant who's having feeding problems (Bertini, Dani, Trochini & Rubaltelli, 2001). Therefore, the decline in bilirubin levels has more to do with receiving frequent and adequate intake of calories from the infant formula than the breastmilk causing the elevated levels of bilirubin. In most cases when breastfed infants are shown to have elevated bilirubin levels, mothers are encouraged to discontinue breastfeeding and encouraged to begin the use of infant formula. This solution is routinely offered by health care professionals instead of working to correct the breastfeeding management problems which will result in an increase in caloric intake and a decline in bilirubin levels.

For many of the misconceptions that have surfaced throughout the years, many of them take their origin with misinformation received from physicians and health care providers, family members and friends. A great many health care providers: primary care physicians, pediatrician and others admit that they feel ill prepared with regard to breastfeeding knowledge and management skills (Freed et al., 1995). This should not be a surprise when during their residency trainings a great many physicians do not receive any technical training on breastfeeding techniques or curriculum training in human lactation. Another important aspect that greatly perpetuates misconceptions about breastfeeding is the attitudes that physicians have regarding the benefits of breastfeeding. Many physicians do not agree or are unconvinced that the research that surrounds the many short and long term benefits of breastfeeding and the use of human milk for infants is true. These attitudes and perceptions are passed along to patients through verbal gestures, a reluctance to declare breastfeeding as the optimal feeding choice or through the use of literature endorsing infant formula products.

There are many policies in place which also perpetuate many misconceptions regarding breastfeeding. The current policy of early discharge for mothers and infants undermine the breastfeeding process. Although the breastfeeding act is one that is very natural, the process of breastfeeding takes effort, education and support to foster an environment for successful breastfeeding. The optimal time to receive the initial instruction on breastfeeding is immediately after delivery of shortly thereafter. However many mothers are discharged within 24-48 hours of delivery, which leaves little time for breastfeeding education. This does not allow for education, instruction and follow-up on proper breastfeeding management. The current recommendation of American Academy of Pediatrics is that newborns discharged at less than 48 hours of age be seen within 2-3 days of discharge. More recent recommendations regarding breastfeeding is that "formal evaluation of breastfeeding performance.... be undertaken during the first 24 to 48 hours after delivery and again at the early follow-up visit, which should occur 48 to 72 hours after discharge (Gartner & Lee, 1999).

Chapter 2

Times Ain't Like They Used To Be

Throughout history breastfeeding has been apart of the African American experience. During slavery African American women served as wet nurses for the children of the plantation owners as well as nursing their own children. Historically, feeding practices up through the 19th and 20th century included breastfeeding well into the second year of life (Calamoro, 2000). Consequently, in the late 1930s the Council of the American Medical Association began indicating that strained fruit and vegetables should be fed to infants at about 4 to 6 months (Bronner et al., 1999). This recommendation along with other key factors parallels the decline that was seen in the 1930s and subsequent years of all infants being exclusively breastfed for up to a year or longer.

The infant feeding practices of African Americans have been rooted in family tradition. In traditional Africa it has been the custom since the beginning of time for mothers to breastfeed their infants and to do so openly, and in public. Unfortunately, with the influence from the western world, along with the saturation of infant formula into developing countries, the attitudes regarding breastfeeding are shifting. Since those days when it was culturally acceptable for African American women to breastfed their infants and up until the 21st century, there has been a total shift in the perception and attitudes surrounding the role that breastfeeding should play as part of the nutrition for African American infants.

For many generations African Americans and particularly for African American women, religion and their spirituality has been a guiding force for their lives. The bible makes reference to the importance of the suckling experience and that for the mother it should take precedent over anything else. Moses, who was rescued from the Nile River by the sister of Pharaoh, was given over immediately to the nurse (who was actually his biological mother) so that he might suckle. Only after he had been weaned was he given back to the sister of Pharaoh.

Hannah who could not conceive a child prayed to God and asked that she may bare a son. She went on to say that if this request were granted she would give the son back to God. God granted Hannah's request and she bore a son Samuel. Only after Hannah had weaned Samuel did she take him to the temple and give him back to God. This act shows the significance of the suckling experience. Samuels suckling experience with his mother took precedent over the promise that had been made to God.

We find ourselves in an era where for many it is culturally unacceptable for African Americans to breastfed. Although the breastfeeding rates are increasing, some look upon breastfeeding as an unnecessary act, and one without much merit. Mothers that choose to breastfed are asked to validate their reasons as to why they would opt to breastfeed as apposed to using formula. For those who are around the mother that is breastfeeding, many seem uneasy and unsure as to where to turn their head as if a shameful act is taking place. The changing perceptions surrounding breastfeeding did not happen just by chance. There were many direct and indirect forces that altered our attitudes regarding a practice that has been apart of our culture since the beginning of time.

Wet-Nursing

Wet-nursing, the act of breastfeeding an infant that is not yours, was first used by the middle and upper class as an alternative feeding method. They considered breastfeeding to be animal like and many had the economic resources to utilize alternative feeding methods. Physicians in the late 19th century and at the turn of the century greatly believed in the benefits of breastfeeding. They sought the employment of wet-nurses for well-to-do families. Wet-nursing was greatly associated with the lower class and the women that accepted positions as wet-nurses were poor and in desperate need. There was great controversy surrounding the use of African American women as wet-nurses. Physicians and families seeking wet-nurses oftentimes questioned the ability of the African American women's body to produce a quality milk that would be beneficial to babies (Woof, 1999). African American women were chosen as wet-nurses when no other suitable wet-nurse could be found.

In the early 20th century fewer and fewer women were becoming wet nurses. The negative connotations associated with the profession along with the small wages paid decreased the number of available wet nurses. At this time physicians still believed that human milk was the best source of nutrients for infants, especially those who were premature and suffering from other ailments. They responded by organizing human milk stations for the sale of bottled breastmilk. They felt that there would be fewer objections to the donor milk because an infant would not have to actually suckle for the "lower class" wet nurse but would still be receiving the benefits of human milk. Again controversy arose when African American women began donating their milk. Objections were so great, that bureaus stop accepting breastmilk from African American women. When donor milk was accepted from African American women it was pooled with the milk of white mothers.

26

Influence from the Medical Profession

Most of the infants born in the United States in the late 19th and early 20th century did not take place in the hospital. In the rural south where most African Americans resided during this time, there were many barriers that inhibited them from utilizing traditional medicine. One of the biggest reasons was financial; most African Americans did not have the resources to utilize hospitals. Therefore it was a common practice for African American infants to be delivered at home. Midwives attended to the births within the African American community. Most of the midwives were African American and lived in the communities in which they served. The use of midwives had a positive influence on African American mothers and their choosing to breastfeed. Many midwives believed that breastmilk carried special powers for the baby and because the midwives were trusted in the communities the mothers embraced the knowledge that they shared. The use of midwives help to strengthen and preserve the traditions related to childbirth in the African American community and breastfeeding was directly associated with childbirth. The midwives also served as the "lactation consultants" as they are now called, and was able to share the how –to regarding the act of breastfeeding based on the many experiences that they had encountered. There were other benefits that mothers received from having at-home births. At-home births allowed mother and baby to immediately bond after delivery and to have breastfeeding start immediately after delivery, which is an important component of successful breastfeeding. Delivering at home also allowed other mothers and female relatives an opportunity to be apart of the birthing process by which they were able to share the information on the how-to of breastfeeding. Back during those times, breastfeeding an infant was just an extension of the childbirth process and generations of women and men were able to witness mothers actively participating in breastfeeding without any degree of shame. This created a social acceptance of breastfeeding. However there was a gradual shift in the acceptance of breastfeeding as the social dynamics of the African American community changed.

Sharecropping was the way of life for most African Americans in the rural south during those times. This work required the mothers to work in the fields as well as the men. In addition to the work in the fields, mothers cared for their babies. African American mothers found innovative ways to continue to provide their infants with nourishment through breastfeeding while continuing to work in the field. Many of the mothers would come together working in the same field and put their infants under a shade tree. Periodically the mothers would come in and check on the babies and feed them and go back to the field (Personal Communication, Rena Mae Purnell, 1999). African American mothers were very resourceful and had to be creative in their supplemental feeding practices. Mothers at that time believe greatly in the benefits of breastfeeding, however there were times when they would need to provide their babies with another feeding option other than breast milk. These mothers would make what was known as a "sugar tiddy." This "sugar tiddy" was made by taking a cloth and forming it into the shape of a breast and saturating it with sugar and butter (Personal Communication, Mattie Norwood, 2001). The infants would suck on this "sugar tiddy" as a pacifier or alternative feeding until the mother was able to provide the infant with breastmilk. This was an innovative way of providing a breast milk substitute for the infants that did not interfere with the breastfeeding process as does many of the commercial breastfeeding substitutes that are available today.

The Great Migration, the termed used to describe the huge number of African Americans moving from the rural south to the cities of the north during and after World War II resulted in a shift in many of the social behaviors that had traditionally been apart of the African American community. One area that has had direct and indirect affects on the rates in which African American women initiated breastfeeding was the increased number of female-headed households, and the increase in single motherhood within the African American community. After 1960, the prevalence of children living with two-parents dropped from 72 % to 59 % in 1970. By 1990, only 33 % of African American children in northern cities were living with two parents (Tolnay, 1997). The prevalence of single motherhood doubled in the African American community from 35 % in 1971 to 69.6 % in 1991(Rendall, 1999).

Women entering into the workforce was another area that affected breastfeeding rates. After the industrial revolution, there was a huge increase in the number of African American women entering into the workforce. During the days of the early 1900s in the rural south, African American women worked primarily as sharecroppers at their homes, as domestics and a few were able to secure jobs as teachers. The move north offered African American women access to jobs and trades that had not been available to them in the south. In 1940, 37.8% of African American women were in the work force (Coleman, 2000). This number does not account for the number of African American women who were working as domestics. At those times the census statistics were not including domestic workers in their count. The Equal Pay Act of 1963 was passed which ended discrimination of less pay for women for similar jobs as men, along with The Civil Rights movement of 1964 or Title VII which outlawed discrimination in hiring based on race religion or sex which helped to bring about a change in hiring practices. With this new liberation in the workplace, breastfeeding was being considered to be restrictive and confining and a barrier to the new independence that African

American women were experiencing. During this time of shifting social dynamics within the African American community, commercial infant formula was being marketed as a convenient alternative to breastfeeding, especially for the working mother.

As traditional medicine was becoming the norm, many began to question the effectiveness of midwives and home deliveries. Although the research studies show that between 1930 and 1960, hospitals births attributed to more birth injuries and obstetric mortality than home births, and that home births were not less safe than hospital births (Devitt, 1977). Before 1930 all hospital cost were paid out of pocket which made it difficult for most African Americans to utilize traditional medicine. In the late 1930s the Blue Cross Association was formed which allowed for medical services to be paid by the organization and in exchange the insurer paid small monthly fees. In 1943, the Emergency Maternal and Infant Care (EMIC) program was developed. This program offered medical care to the wives of the soldiers. By 1950, 51% of civilians had insurance for hospitalization, which made hospital births more accessible and affordable (O'Mara, 1998). In 1935, 37 % of births took place in hospitals, by 1960 it had increased to 97% and by 1970, 99.4% of all births took place in the hospital (Devitt, 1977). This transition to hospital births had a huge impact on the rate in which African American mothers initiated breastfeeding. At one point only the middle and upper class were using hospitals for childbirth. In 1946, congress passed the Hill-Burton Act, which allocated $4 billion to build and modernize hospitals. By 1966 some 4,700 hospitals were built or improved using these funds. The Hill–Burton money was use to build eighty-nine segregated hospitals in the south and facilities in the north that had segregation policies that inhibited African Americans from utilizing them, although these facilities were oftentimes in the African American community (Garret, 2000 p.325).

When hospital deliveries were made available to African American mothers they greatly embraced this practice believing it was a step up and the entryway to a pain free delivery. Between 1959 and 1965, all but 26% of African American mothers who delivered their babies in hospitals were anesthetized (Rooks, 1997 p 53). During this time "twilight sleep" was the term used to describe the anesthesia process. It was a combination of morphine used to control the pain, and scopolamine, an amnesiac that caused the mother to have no memory of giving birth (Wright, 2001; Rook, 1997 p. 22). With the increased use of anesthesia by African American women and many other factors, the control that African American mothers once had over their own childbirth experiences were now being controlled by physicians, insurance companies and hospitals. This shift in control would have huge impacts on the rates in which African American women initiated breastfeeding.

In the early part of the 20th century hospitals maintained formula laboratories on-site to prepare infant formula for newborns and other formula-fed infants (Formon, 2001). From an economic standpoint hospitals found it to be more cost effective to purchase ready-to-feed infant formula from commercial suppliers and they slowly discontinued their on-site production of infant formula. This shift started the trend of competition among commercial suppliers for hospital infant formula contracts. It also set the stage for price and cost to be the determining factor of which infant formula was chosen or used for a hospital as opposed to the best products for the particular needs of the infant. As the infant formula industry grew, hospitals and physicians began entering into contracts with the infant formula manufacturers and they began exclusively endorsing particular brands of infant formula, and utilizing this formula on their maternity wards. This embracement of infant formula by the medical profession was one key change that started the societal shift from a

31

breastfeeding society to a bottle-friendly society. The psychology of this trend was the bottle-feeding was associated with being urbanized and sophisticated, and breastfeeding was associated with being poor and old-fashioned.

Hospital births also started the trend of separating mother and infant. The term called rooming in was not practiced. In 1960, practically no United States hospital had rooming in or allowed mothers and babies to remain together after delivery (Latham, 1998). This practice was the direct opposite of what was traditionally practiced within the African American community under the care of the midwives. This separation of mother and baby decreased the likely-hood that the mother would be able to successfully breastfeed her infant. The practice of infants being kept on maternity wards facilitated a standard practice of feeding them formula and/or glucose water, which also impacted the success of mothers initiating breastfeeding. This shift is yet another example of the transfer of control that took place regarding infant feeding when African American mothers began to utilized hospitals for childbirth.

The medical profession together with the FDA and pharmaceutical companies with their combined forces, had another impact on breastfeeding rates with the 1980 approval of the drug Parlodel (bromocriptine) for the use as post-partum lactation suppression, or in other words, to dry up breast milk and prevent breast engorgement. Many consumer advocates and medical professionals argued that bromocriptine was too dangerous of a drug to be used in this capacity. So after years of disputes, the FDA called for all United States pharmaceutical companies to voluntarily stop marketing bromocriptine for lactation suppression. All the pharmaceutical companies complied with the FDA's request except Sandoz Company. A lawsuit was filed against the FDA by the Public Citizen

32

Health Research Group and the National Women's Health Network to force the FDA to rescind its approval of bromocriptine for lactation suppression (McCarthy, 1994). It took just one day after the lawsuit was filed for the FDA to remove its approval of bromocriptine, and one day after that for the Sandoz Company to agree to stop marketing bromocriptine as use for lactation suppression. The lawsuit stated that the FDA had received 531 reports of adverse reactions in young and middle-aged women who had taken bromocriptine including strokes, heart attacks, severe hypertension and seizures. Thirty-two women died and many more were severely disabled as a result of this drug (McCarthy, 1994). The unfortunate aspect of the issue is that doctors are still able to prescribe and utilize bromocriptine for use as lactation suppression because the drug is still on the market and used to treat various health conditions including Parkinson's disease.

Most hospitals, and many within the medical profession do not support a positive breastfeeding environment there will always be a perceived need for lactation suppression drugs. It is ironic that hospitals through their practices actually create environments that fosters the assumed need for lactation suppression drugs: giving infants formula or glucose water as a standard practice, the separation of mother and baby, by not sharing with mothers the many benefits of breastfeeding and overall not encouraging mothers to breastfeed. It is interesting that the medical profession and the pharmaceutical companies were able to come up a medical solution for the problem of women not breastfeeding. A medical problem was established, a diagnosis made and a drug treatment was provided to a problem that really wouldn't require a medial solution if mothers were supported and encouraged to breastfeed. So actually the pharmaceutical companies created a product and then the medical profession and hospitals with their many barriers to successful breastfeeding helps maintain a market for that product. The result is that the mothers who were given, and possible are given this drug for lactation suppression risk serious health complication and possibly death, and the many infants who could have been the recipients of the benefits of breast milk, were not or will not be, all because of potential profits to be made by the distribution of this drug treatment for the assumed medical problem.

In the late 1950s and early 1960s there was a trend reversal to a more natural childbirth experience. Baby boomers and the white middle-class began to denounce the use of anesthesia and began to re-embrace breastfeeding. The Lamaze technique was beginning to be used in the United States to control pain during delivery, and the La Leche League was formed in Chicago dedicated to promoting and providing support groups for breastfeeding mothers. During this time African American women began to increase their usage of infant formula, emulating the earlier mothering styles of the middle class, something they had not been able to afford before the war (Golden, 1996).

In the early 1960s, President Lyndon Johnson's War on Poverty greatly impacted the availability of health services within the African American community. The income supplement program Aid to Families with Dependent Children (ADFC) was established in 1960 and the Medicaid and Medicare programs were established in 1965, which provided health insurance for poor and disabled individuals. These programs allowed many African Americans access to health services that had not been available to them in the past. Before 1966, and the passing of Medicare and Medicaid, African Americans rarely saw doctors. After 1966, the poor and African Americans were actually visiting doctors more frequently than whites (Garrett, 2000 p.

346). This shift provided physicians with an opportunity to exert a greater control on the infant feeding practices of African Americans.

In response to the high infant mortality rate and the high rates of iron deficiency among low-income populations, the Special Supplemental Nutrition Program WIC was established in 1972. This program provided it participants' vouchers for free infant formula and food. There is a great debate as to whether or not the development of the WIC program and the distribution of free infant formula have negatively impacted the breastfeeding rates within the African American community. Although the written policy of the WIC program is to promote breastfeeding as the best way to feed an infant, the general consensus is that WIC is a program that disseminates free infant formula. In 1993, the WIC program provided $500 million for formula purchase and distribution, and only 8 million for the support of breastfeeding (Schwab, 1996). The infants who are participants of the WIC program experience the highest rates of morbidity and mortality and would benefit most from breastfeeding. However mothers with lower incomes are less likely to initiate and continue breastfeeding. A 1997 study by the Department of Agriculture found that 31% of WIC mothers initiated breastfeeding, but only 16 % were still breastfeeding at five months (Kaufman, 1999). The data shows that from 1984 through 1989, women who were African American, younger, had not more than a high school diploma, or enrolled in the WIC program were less likely to be breastfeeding their infant at six months (Wright, 2001).

There has been resurgence in the number of African American women breastfeeding, but it is far below the rates of Whites and Latino mothers. The African American breastfeeding rates have not recovered from the many historical influences and barriers that have inhibited African Americans from breastfeeding. To combat many of the barriers that exist in the hospital setting against mother's breastfeeding, UNICEF and the World Health Organization (WHO) has established the Baby Friendly Hospital Initiative (BFHI). With this initiative hospitals sign contracts stating that their hospital will no longer be a source of misinformation regarding breastfeeding, and the practices that they promote in the hospital will be ones which create an environment for the mother and the baby to participate in the breastfeeding process. Many physicians admit that they do not feel adequately trained to provide breastfeeding information to mothers who may be interested. In addition they routinely disseminate literature that explains and support the use of infant formula. The various medical associations must take a stand and insist that human lactation and breastfeeding training become apart of the overall curriculum for physicians, nurses and other health care professionals who work directly with mothers and babies.

Throughout history there has been negative social stigmas associated with breastfeeding. This practice has been commonly linked with the poor, those of lower socioeconomic status and those who lived in non-urbanized communities. Since the beginning of time there has been a cloud of doubt hanging over the heads of African American women regarding the quality of their breastmilk, and its ability to serve as the primary nutrients for the development of their infants. While African American mothers served as wet nurses for others, many African American babies died as a result of not receiving breastmilk. The attitudes, perceptions and misconceptions surrounding breastfeeding have been apart of the African American experience since the beginning of time. These negative attitudes have been passed down from generation to generation, along with the subliminal messages that are sent throughout society from health care professionals, infant formula manufacturers, the mass media and others regarding the quality and quantity of breastmilk produced by African American women has impacted the rates in which African American women chose breastfeeding as the sources of their infant's nutrition.

We are still today suffering from clouds of doubt regarding our ability to effectively feed our infants so that they might grow and thrive. In this new millennium we have few role models when looking for others who have breastfed their infants. There are generations of women who have never seen or heard of anyone in their family who has breastfed or have been breastfed. This generation also includes men who were never breastfed, or have seen a women around them in the breastfeeding process and as a result they offer little support or actual discourage breastfeeding. The lack of support and discouragement towards breastfeeding has been key to the low rates in which African Americans participate in the breastfeeding process.

African Americans, who were courted and romanced into the use of traditional medicine, find themselves looking at other ethnicities utilizing a childbirth experience that they relied on out of necessity that now today is being characterized as natural. As a result of the dysfunctional relationship that African Americans have with the medical profession and insurance companies, it seems as if it would be impossible to severe this relationship and rekindle a healthier relationship. And because breastfeeding is so closely associated with the childbirth experience, and because it is all in some way or another tied to profits, it would seem to reason that the initiation of breastfeeding and breastfeeding rates within the African American community would continue to suffer as a result of this dysfunctional relationship.

There are many direct and indirect factors that have influenced the rate in which African American women initiate breastfeeding.

Although, many believe that their choices as to how they will feed their infant is an independent one and solely based on the present tense, there is a great deal of history and influences that has shaped the attitudes and opinions regarding infant feeding choices within the African American community.

Chapter 3

Human Milk, it does a Body Good

In this day and age if you used the phrase "Human Milk" many people will not know what you are referring to. It is also true that many do not recognize that out of the act of breastfeeding, infants actually receive human milk. In reproduction the female can participate in three components: becoming pregnant, giving birth and providing nutrients. Unfortunately within the African American community, we have in great numbers disassociated ourselves with the third component which is commonly known as breastfeeding.

Humans are considered to be mammals, which means that we are warm-blooded animals who have the ability to feed our young. All mammals, human and animals, have the organs and the hormones, the anatomy and physiology to allow them to nurture their young in this way (Latham, 1998). Human beings are set apart from other animals because of our cognitive and intellectual capacity. With our intellect, cognitive capacity and now technology, the role that human milk should play in the development of the human body has been questioned and greatly diminished. Many have accepted our many advances in medicine and technology in the field of infant nutrition to be equivalent or superior to the human milk that is produce through the act of breastfeeding.

Alternative feeding methods have been used throughout history. The focus for the most part has been on the nutritional aspects of human milk. Commercial infant formula was greatly embraced because it was marketed as a nutritional improvement over human milk.

Human milk however can no longer be considered just for its nutritional aspects. In the last decade there has been a great deal of research done on the non-nutritional components of human milk. This research has set human milk apart from all other infant feeding methods, and has made it impossible for it to be duplicated. Unfortunately this information about all the benefits of human milk have been reported in medical journals and throughout academia, but has not trickled down to the mothers and those who are making decisions as to how they will feed their infants.

For centuries even dating back to the Stone Age the benefits of human milk in fighting infections have been known. In the United States and in other developed countries it is perceived that many of the infections and diseases that plague developing countries are no longer prevalent or dangerous to developed societies. The prevalence of certain illnesses and diseases may be less common in the United States and other developed countries, but infants are still at risk because of their immature and underdeveloped immune systems. We are entering into a very frightening public health era, we now find that there are strains of bacteria that are resistance to the drugs that we currently have available. Many scientist, pharmaceutical companies and others with vested interest are looking to the development of new antibodies and other drugs to combat this problem without much exploration of the role that human milk can play. One example of this is the 1998 FDA approval of RotaShield, a vaccine for rotavirus, the leading cause of diarrhea in children. The vaccine was suspended because it caused many cases of bowel obstruction in infants (Child vaccine, 1999). More and more research has been conducted in the area of rotavirus. Rotavirus is considered to be a serious health problem in both developing and developed countries. Lactadherin a milk sugar that is a component of human milk acts as a decoy for the rotavirus in the intestines of the breastfed infant. The rotavirus attaches to the lactadherin instead of an actual cell, and is flushed from the intestines of the breastfed infant (Seppa, 1998). As a result, breastfed infants are less likely to develop the rotavirus infection and if contracted, symptoms are less severe as compared to formula-fed infants (Newburg, 1997).

Human milk has an abundant supply of various protective components. The immature immune and GI of infants predispose them to the development of infections during the first year of life. The non-nutritional proteins of human milk act together to provide protection to the breastfed infant against potential invaders of their bodies. These include Secretory Immonoglobin A (IgA), Lactoferrin, Lysozyme and many other factors. IgA stands out because of its specific association with maternal antibodies that the mother has built throughout her life. The mother produces specific IgA antigens to which she and the infant has been exposed. The antigens that have been taken in by the mother are recognized and a resistance is built up against these antigens. This recognition and antibodies resistance against these antigens is passed on to the infant through the mother's milk. Specific IgA's work to protect the immature gastrointestinal tract of the infant from those antigens. Human milk colostrum, the first milk secreted after delivery, contains more than 1g/l of IgA and the fully breastfed infant receives about 1 gram a day of IgA (Weaver, Arthur, Bunn, & Thomas, 1997).

There are more than 300 milk sugars in human milk, and many of the roles of these milk sugars have yet to be uncovered. One milk sugar in particular that have been receiving a great deal of attention is oligosaccharides. Oligosaccharides, is the third largest component of human milk after lactose and fat, and is considered to be one of the primary reasons breastfed infants are able to resist infections. It is thought that oligosaccharides actually serve as decoys for pathogens that try to invade the body of the infant. When the pathogens attempt to invade the cells of the infant, the pathogen attaches itself to the oligosaccaride or another milk sugar decoy that is not attached to an actual cell of the infant (Newburg, 1997). This is important because in order for the pathogen to invade the body of an infant, it must first attach itself and cause infection, and there must to be an environment for which the bacteria can attach itself to the cell. So in actuality, the oligosaccarides and the other milk sugars serve as gatekeepers working to keep invaders outs. Oligosaccarides are found in limited amounts in infant formula and cow's milk (Brand & McVeagh, 1999).

Prebotics is a term used to describe factors that are found in human milk which stimulate the growth of good bacteria within the intestines. Bifidobacteria is a bacterium that is receiving a great deal of attention. Breastfed infants have a higher concentration of bifidobacterium in their stool and intestines than formula-fed infants, or infants who are fed mixed diets (Newburg, 1997; Bezkorovainy, 2001). It accounts for 95 % of the "good bacteria" in the colon of a breastfed infant (Macfarlane & Cummings, 1999). The growth of bifidobacterium thrives in human milk (Tram-Hunter, 1996). The components that are needed to stimulate the growth of bifidobacterium are found in all human milk but are absent from cow's milk, which would also make it absent from infant formula (Newburg, 1997).

Another unique aspect of human milk is its ability to adapt to the specific developmental needs of an infant. This aspect of human milk is all so often understated, underrated and very much downplayed when comparisons are made to infant formula. Colostrum, which is the first fluid produced by the mother after delivery is rich in antibodies, high in protein and low in fat.

Colostrum contains higher levels of many nutrients and protective agents. Colostrum might also be considered the first immunization that the breastfed infant receives. After several days of producing colostrum, it is replaced with transitional milk, and then with mature milk. Mature milk is higher in fat, but lower in protein and antibodies. Throughout the suckling experience the fat content of human milk gradually changes. The first milk ingested has a lower fat content which is called the fore milk. As the suckling continues the fat content increases and this is called the hind milk (Wagner &Anderson, 1996). The increased fat content of hind milk facilitates satiety in the infant. Unlike human milk, infant formula is always the same and never changing, it does not, and cannot, meet the specific developmental needs of a growing infant.

Another exciting aspect of human milk that many seem not to give much thought to, or may not even know, is that the breastfed infant has the opportunity to experience a variety of tastes and smells. Again, unlike infant formula which is constant in its taste and smell, the taste and smell of human milk is influenced by the diet of the mother (Winberg & Porter, 1998). This early introduction to varied tastes and smells allows for the stimulation of the sensory systems of the breastfed infant.

Composition

Protein
The protein content of human milk is specifically designed to meet the growth needs of a developing human infant. Protein provides 7% of the calories in human milk compared to 20% of the calories in cow's milk. The protein of milk is broken down into two categories: casein and whey. Human milk protein is predominately whey, and it

has a whey- to-casein ratio of 60:40. Cow's milk has an 80 casein to 20 whey ratio. Whey proteins are easier for the infant to digest, it contains various growth factors, increases iron absorption, and helps to break down lactose, which is the primary carbohydrates in human milk (Tigges, 1997). Casein proteins form hard curds in the stomach of an infant and are harder for them to digest. Since human milk is considered to be the gold standard for infant nutrition, infant formula manufacturers try to model their product after human milk. Although they admit that it is impossible to replicate human milk, protein is the area that they attempt to try. In an effort to mimic the whey to casein ratio found in human milk, infant formula manufacturers use demineralized whey powder and whey protein that has been extracted during cheese making and add it to their infant formula mix. Because this increases the amount of whey in their product, it is marketed that the protein content of infant formula is "close to that of mothers milk." This is misleading for consumers. Also the whey composition of human milk and cow's milk is very different. The bulk of the whey composition of human milk is made up of x-lactalbumin and lactoferrin. The whey composition of cow's milk is made up of b-lactoglobulin and x-lactalbumin. Human milk does not contain b-lactalbumin. Therefore because of the significant differences in the whey composition of human and cow's milk, they cannot and do not produce the same results (Rolf, Maise, Maynard & Secretin, 1999). Another aspect about the whey to casein ratio of human milk is that it is not constant. During early infancy human milk has a whey to casein ratio of 90:10, mature milk has a range of 60:40 and the ratio after 8 months of breastfeeding is approximately 50:50 (Tigges, 1997). So the claims made by the infant formula manufacturers may be true but they are deceptive and misleading and void of the entire truth. A perfect example of this is the claims made by Nestle' about the Carnation Good Start infant formula. The advertisements states that this formula contains 100% whey proteins, and because of that they can say that their product has "comfort proteins" that are easier for the infant to digest, just like those found in human milk." As stated above, yes this product does contain 100% whey protein, but it is not the same as the whey protein found in human milk, it has a totally different whey composition. But to look at their advertisements, one would believe that the Carnation Good Start Infant formula is the same, or an even better product than human milk, based on the 100% whey composition.

Source	Protein Level
Human Milk/ Early Lactation	10-12g/l
Human Milk/ Mature Milk	8-9g/l
Cow' based Infant Formula	15-16g/l
Soy based Infant Formula	19-22g/l

Table 1 Nutritional aspects of soy formula (Lonnerdal, 1994).

	Whey	Casein
Human Milk	60	40
Cow's Milk	20	80
Similac	18	82
Gerber	18	82
Enfamil	60	40
SMA	60	40
Carnation Good Start	100	

Table 2 Whey: Casein compositions of common formulas. Adapted from Wagner, 1996.

Amino Acid

The amino acid content of human milk is also specific to support the growth of a human infant. There are several amino acids that vary greatly in their quantity in human milk. The differences between human milk and cow's milk amino acid profile are quite distinct. Human milk has high levels of cystein and low levels of methonine, and the opposite is true for cow's milk which has a higher content of methonine and lower levels of cystein. Cystein is needed to for the development of the infant's central nervous system. Methonine and phenylalanine, which are the primary amino acids in cow's milk is difficult for infant bodies to break down because they lack the cysthionine enzyme in the liver to do so. Another important amino acid is taurine, is needed for bile salt formation and for visual and brain function is found naturally in human milk. Cow's milk does not contain taurine, therefore it is added to infant formula.

Tryptophan

Tryptophan (Trp) is an amino acid that has a large role in infant nutrition. Trp is important to the neurobehavioral development of an infant. It has a significant role in the maturing of the brain, helping to regular food intake, signaling to the infant that they are satisfied and have had enough to eat, and the regulation of the sleep-wake rhythm (Heine, 1999). Human milk is a rich source of Trp. Approximately 2.2-2.4 % of human milk is Trp and colostrum contains the highest levels (Heine, 1999). Cow's milk contains only1.3 % Trp. As a result of the low levels of Trp found in cow's milk, infant formula is low in Trp as well. To increase the amount of Trp in infant formula the protein levels are increased well above the levels found in human milk. This presents several problems because with the higher protein levels, other amino acids compete with the Trp for absorption, and as a result formula fed infant may not be receiving adequate amounts of Trp (Heine, 1999).

Carbohydrate

The primary ingredient of human milk is lactose. Lactose is the main source of energy for the infant. Carbohydrates provide 40% of the calories of human milk compared to 30% from cow's milk. To closer resemble human milk, carbohydrate supplements are added to infant formula to make up for the inadequacy of the carbohydrate level when compared to human milk.

Fats

Both human milk and cow's milk is made up of 50% fat. However the composition of that fat is very different. The fat of human milk is made up of medium-chain triglycerides and monosaturated fats and cow's milk is basically saturated, short and long chained fatty acids. Human milk also contains a greater amount of the enzyme lipase, which works to increase the amount of fat that is absorbed (Tigges, 1997). The triglyceride structure of human milk fat plays an important role in its digestibility and this cannot be duplicated in infant formula (Benson & Masor, 1994).

Cholesterol is the fat that is considered to be taboo for adults because a high level of cholesterol is associated with an increased risk for the development of cardiovascular disease. Cholesterol is however needed for the growing infant. Human milk has an abundant supply of cholesterol 115-150mg/l, compared to infant formula which has one-third of the amount found in human milk (Katoku, Yamanda, Kuwata & Tamotsu, 1996).

Vitamins and Minerals

The vitamin and mineral composition of human milk is unique to the species. Human milk has a low concentration of various vitamins and minerals but a high absorption rate when compared to the vitamins and minerals found in cow's milk and infant formula, particularly iron, calcium and zinc (Lonnerdale, 1996). The sodium, chloride, potassium, calcium and phosphate levels in cow's milk are double and often times triple the level found in human milk. The higher amounts that are found in cow's milk and infant formula place a great deal of stress on the kidneys of the infant.

Human Milk and Cognitive Development
Early nutrition is considered to play a role in the cognitive development of an infant. Oftentimes when comparisons are made between breastfed and formula-fed infants the growth, height and weight charts are used to make the comparison. Research is uncovering that the early nutrition of an infant might set the framework for their long-term cognitive development.

Sialic Acid
Sialic acid, a sugar that is derived from oligosaccharides, is found in high concentrations in human milk. These high levels are not found in cow's milk or infant formula. Sialic acid is associated with brain development, cell-to-cell communication and memory (Brand & McVeagh, 1999). Mammals do have the capacity to convert sialic acid from simple sugar, but it is thought that the human infant's liver may not be able to synthesize this process. Research has shown that breastfed infants have two times more sialic acid in their saliva than does formula-fed infants (Tram, 1997). Elephants have high concentrations of sialic acid and elephants are associated with having excellent memories (Brand & McVeagh, 1999).

DHA
DHA, a long-chain polyunsaturated fatty acid that is essential to visual and brain development is considered to play an important role

in the cognitive development of infants. DHA deficiency is associated with visual impairment, learning disabilities, dementia, depression, memory loss and attention-deficit/hyperactivity disorder (ADHD) (Levine, 1998). Human milk is a natural source of DHA. The current infant formula in the United States is not supplemented with DHA and it is thought that the current fatty acid composition of infant formula is not sufficient to allow for the conversion of DHA. Breastfed infants have higher plasma levels of DHA when compared to that of formula-fed infants. Therefore many infants may be at risk for DHA deficiencies. Also preterm infants are at risk for DHA deficiencies because DHA transfer from mother to fetus via the placenta takes place in the last trimester. The DHA content of the fetal brain increases 3-5 times during the final trimester of pregnancy and triples during the first 12 weeks of life (Levine, 1998).

Iron Deficiency
Human milk has a low concentration of iron but as much as 50 % of the iron from human milk is absorbed compared to 7-12 % being absorbed from cow-based infant formula and even less, 1-7 % is absorbed from soy-based infant formula (Iron fortification, 1999). Iron deficiency is associated with measurable lower test scores of motor and mental development and the cognitive damage done by iron deficiency does not appear to be fully irreversible (Raji, 1998). Iron deficiency also increases the tendency of lead to be absorbed (Yip, 1998).

Human Milk and Disease Links
Research is being uncovered everyday regarding the composition of human milk. Infant nutrition is being viewed in a new light based on these research findings. It is being hypothesized that infant nutrition may have long-tem implications in the development of various

chronic diseases and/or other health related problems. The research findings that have been realized for adults are thought to be applicable for infants as well. A good example of this is the role that caratenoids play in the growth and development of the infant, as well as long-term health consequences of them being absent in the diets of infants. Carotenoids are micronutrients that cannot be produced by the human body therefore they must be consumed. Fruits and vegetables are the nature source of carotenoids that humans can consume. Carotenoids have been found to reduce the risk of cancer, cardiovascular disease, age related eye diseases such as cataracts and macular degeneration (Sommerburg et al., 2000). Since infants are unable to consume fruit and vegetables in their early nutrition, the importance of carotenoids in their early diet has not been greatly emphasized until recently. During the prenatal state the fetus received cartoneoids via the placental from the mother. After birth the level of carotenoids decrease or increase depending on the feeding choice. Research has shown that the carotenoid amounts in human milk, greatly differs from that of infant formula. There are over 300 known carotenoids. The one that usually receives the most attention is beta-carotene. This study focused on four of the carotenoids. All of the tested carotenoid was detected in human milk, with the greatest amounts showing up in colostrum. The detectable amounts of carotenoids various infant formulas varied a great deal. In all the formulas tested, the carotenoid levels were at much lower levels than found in human milk (Sommerburg et al., 2000). The amounts were tested at birth and the 2-6th week. The result of this study is significant because it shows an association between infant nutrition and later possible development of diseases. Although there has not been a great deal of work done in the area of carotenoids and newborns, the research does set the stage for a possible link between infant nutrition and development of disease in later life. Also, because this research is in its early stage, the health implications of formula fed newborns having low levels of carotenoids in their body as compared to that of breastfed infants are unknown.

Human Milk, Breastfeeding and Oral Cavity Development
In addition to the many nutritional and protective components of human milk, breastfed infants receive many developmental benefits related to their oral cavity.

The complex act of receiving milk from the breast through suckling by the infant has a positive affect on the development of the oral cavity. When the oral cavity is in its early developmental stage, it is very soft and its shape can be easily altered. The natural shape of an oral cavity is a u-shape. The u-shape allows room for the proper alignment of the teeth. Suckling from the breast is associated with the development of a u-shaped oral cavity. Research has uncovered that during prehistoric times before the invention and widespread use of bottles, and when breastfeeding was the norm, skulls that were examined exhibited characteristics of having U-shaped oral cavities. The more recent skulls showed oral cavities resembling more of V-shapes (Palmer, 1998). The uses of bottles and pacifiers have played a role in the development of the unnatural shape of the oral cavity, most notable into a V-shape. The V-shape of the oral cavity does not support the development of proper alignment of the teeth.

The actual shape of the oral cavity also plays a role in the space that is available for the development of the nasal cavity. This can have an effect on the size of the nasal cavity and impact the effectiveness of breathing. The size and shape of the nasal cavity has also been associated with snoring and obstructive sleep apnea (Palmer, 1998).

Breastfeeding is also associated with the development of normal swallowing. Suckling from the breast as opposed to sucking from a bottle requires totally different mechanics. In order for the breastfed infant to get milk from the breast it requires that they develop a seal around the nipple and areola tissue. Compressing the areola tissue stimulates the release of milk. The tongue action of the breastfed infant is one of a rolling motion. To retrieve the contents of its bottle, the bottle-fed infant's tongue action is more of a piston-like or squeezing motion (Weber, Woodridge & Baum, 1986). The bottle-fed infant has to adapt to the large flow of milk that comes from an artificial nipple by using its tongue. This abnormal motor action of the bottle-fed infant is referred to as a tongue thrust or a deviated swallow. There is a need for greater force to be placed on the artificial nipple to retrieve the contents from the bottle. The forceful pressure that is applied to the artificial nipple causes the cheeks to draw in putting pressure on the gums and teeth. On the other hand, the nipple of a breast is soft and its shape is dictated by the infant's mouth. An artificial nipple is already formed and its shape constant and because there is no standardization for nipple sizes, an infant that uses a variety of nipples will be adjusting and readjusting in an effort to get the content from the bottle.

Breastfeeding is also associated with the development of the mandible and facial muscles. The breastfed infant has to open its mouth wide, move its jaws back and forth and squeeze with the gums to get the milk (Palmer, 1998). The syprahyoid muscle group is responsible for the movement of the jaw back and forth. The suprahyoid groups consist of the digastric, geniohyoid, mylohyoid and stylohyoid muscles. It has been found that the digastic muscle in breastfed infants is two times stronger than in adults to allow for the breastfeeding action (Yasuo, Matsushita, Shinod & Yoshida, 1997). With these muscles working together along with the active tongue and jaw-lowering motion, there is an increase in the suckling strength and development of the muscles (Yasuo et al., 1997).

The development of Baby Bottle Tooth Decay (BBTD) is associated with prolonged and frequent daytime, naptime and nighttime bottle-feeding. It has been suggested that infant formula plays a huge role in the development of BBTD (Erickson, McClintik, Green & LaFleur, 1998). Infant formula, including soy-based has many ingredients that are considered to be cacinogenic: lactose, sucrose, corn syrup solids and glucose polymers (Sleikh, 1996). These carbohydrates in infant formula, along with the bacteria streptococci, come together and form a sticky film on the teeth and over time form cavities (Tinanoff, 1997). There are those that contend that prolonged breastfeeding is also a contributing factor to BBTD. There is an on-going debate as to whether or not breastmilk is carinogenic. Research has concluded that breastmilk is not carinogenic (Erickson & Mazhari, 1999). Unlike infant formula, even when given alone, have ingredients which are cariogenic (Erickson et al, 1998). Not surprisingly in many primitive cultures where breastfeeding was the norm throughout the day and night, for well into the second year of life, the rates of dental cavities in children were extremely low (Erickson et al., 1998). This leads us to believe that human milk is not the enemy that destroys teeth.

Chapter 4

Infant Formula,
What you should know!

The breast-bottle debate has been going for years and will continue throughout this millennium. Unfortunately, the debate has been going on without the entire truth being disclosed to the public. Artificial baby milk was initially developed as a way to feed infants whose mothers had died or abandoned them. Many saw the potential for great profit and the marketing and selling of infant formula began. Infant formula manufacturers have been working hard throughout the decades to convince mothers and society that their product is a perfect alternative to mother's milk. The goal of the infant formula manufacturers is to establish and retain loyal customers and they have several ways of doing this. They give free formula samples to physicians and hospitals to be passed on to the patients, send expectant mothers free gift bags with formula samples to their homes and a host of other marketing techniques to encourage the mother to utilize their products. Hospitals work closely with the infant formula manufacturers and they sign exclusive contracts with them in an agreement to exclusively distribute their particular brand of formula. In exchange, the hospitals receive money, research and educational grants, and many other incentives. The infant formula manufacturers contribute millions of dollars in various forms in an effort to sway the decisions of organizations who are on record as supporting breastfeeding: AAP, The American College of Obstetricians and Gynecologist (ACOG) and the American Medical Association (AMA) (Quick, 1997). The question must be asked, are these professional organizations who have mission statements that declare that they are advocates for maternal and child health issues actually operating in the best interest of the consumers? If a hospital has a contract with a particular brand of infant formula, then that formula is exclusively recommended to their patients. This practice gives an unspoken endorsement from the physician and the hospital as if this brand of formula is the recommended and brand of infant formula. The question that needs to be asked and answered is "would the hospital and/or physician be endorsing this feeding choice if there wasn't a financial incentive to do so? This question, and many more must be asked and answered because these very same medical professionals and health organizations set policies and standards which greatly impact the health and well being of infants.

Composition

Most people probably do not give much thought to the actual ingredients of infant formula. Many will be surprised to learn exactly what the contents are. Milk based infant formulas are made from fat-free cow's milk or a mixture of fat-free cow's milk and partially demineralized whey, a mixture of vegetable oils or vegetable and oleo oils, lactose, vitamins, minerals and taurine (Formon, 1987). Soy-based infant formulas are made from methionine-fortified isolate soy-protein, a mixture of vegetable oils or vegetable and ileo oils, carbohydrates in the form of a cornstarch hydrolysate and/or sucrose, vitamins, minerals, taurine and carnite (Formon, 1987).

There are several other kinds of infant formula that are marketed as specialized infant formula. The two primary types are casein-hydrolysated or whey-hydrolysated. With casein-hydrolysated formula, the casein levels are broken down into smaller parts and the thought is that it will be less of problem for the infant to digest. It has been stated that casein hydrolysated formula tends to have a bitter taste and be very expensive compared to Whey-hydrolysated formula which does not require as must processing as casein-hydrolysated formula and it is said to taste better and be less expensive.

Processing

Infant formula must go through a great deal of processing to get to the point where the infant can consume it. Infant formula is heat-treated in an effort to maintain the bacteriologic quality of the product, to assure that the nutrients are properly mixed, and to reduce the curd tension from the cow's milk casein protein (Cook, 1989; Lonnerdale & Hernell, 1998). There are several ways that the heating of infant formula can take place: Resort Sterilization, High Temperature Short-Time, or Ultrahigh Temperature. To produce the powdered form of infant formula spray drying is required as an additional step beyond the heat treatment.

The processing technique that is chosen can affect of the digestibility or the stability of the content. For example, protein digestibility is higher in infant formula that has been heat treated by ultra high temperatures over that of resort sterilization (Lonnerdale & Hernell, 1998). Unfortunately, infant formula is not labeled as to how it was processed, as with other areas of infant formula production, the consumers must rely on the infant formula manufacturers to operate in their best interest.

Soy

Soy protein is the cheapest source of protein and has been used as a substitute for cow's milk since the turn of the century (Essex, 1996). Forty percent of all infants fed infant formula will be given soy formula in their first year of life (Lonnerdale, Jayawickrama & Lien, 1999). Many physicians prescribe the use of soy infant formula when an infant is thought to be allergic to cow's milk or have some type of gastrointestinal problem. The carbohydrate composition of soy-based infant formula is sucrose and corn syrup, and many of the minerals in soy-based infant formula are not absorbed efficiently (Stehlin, 1996).

Several organizations have called for the removal of soy infant formula from the market, recommending it be used only under prescription, and that it should carry a warning label (Soy infant, 1999). There are several potential problems with the use of soy-based infant formula:

- Infants that use soy-based infant formula are at increased risk of thyroid disorder. They are two to three times more likely to develop thyroid disease than if they were drinking cow-based infant formula or human milk (Kerlin, 1999).

- The protein content of soy-based infant formula is much higher than human milk and cow-based infant formula. (See Table 1)

- Soy-based infant formula contains phytate, a group of plant substances not found in human milk. The absorption of the trace element zinc is greatly reduced by the phytates in soy-based infant formula. Approximately 60% of zinc is absorbed from human milk compared to 25% from soy-based infant formula (Lonnerdale & Hernell, 1998).

- Soy also contains high amounts of phytoestrogen. Phytoestrogens are endocrine disruptors. Infants fed soy-based infant formula have phytoestrogen levels of 13,000 to

22,000 times higher than normally found in an infant's body (Walker, 2000). Phytoestrogens can create a steroid hormone imbalance and can affect sex organ function. The phyoestrogen level in a days worth of soy-based infant formula is equal to the amount found in five birth control pills (Soy infant, 1999).

- The manganese levels found in soy-based infant formula is extremely high in comparison to human milk and cow-based infant formula. There is an extremely high retention rate of manganese in infancy. The retention of manganese could result in manganese toxicity of the brain, which is where a large portion of absorbed manganese is retained (Lonnerdale & Hernell, 1989).

Many people are jumping on the soy bandwagon. As people are becoming more health conscious they are looking for ways to consume diets that will reduce their risk for disease and other health complications. Consumer interest has been further peaked with the use of soy since the FDA's approval of soy to carry the heart health claim. Soy is a very abundant crop in the United States and is a multibillion-dollar industry. The soy industry is constantly looking to find other avenues in which to utilize this abundant product, and infant formula is just one of many.

More than half of the soybean crop is genetically modified. This means that the DNA of the beans has been altered in some way. In a consumer report test, three soy-based infant formulas tested positive for having genetically modified ingredients: Enfamil ProSobee, Similac Isomil and Nestle Carnation Alsoy (Genetically Engineered, 1999). Scientist, special interest groups and others are debating whether or not the use of genetically modified foods poses risks to humans. Unlike other countries, genetically modified foods are not required to carry labels in the Unites States. The infants who are consuming soy-based infant formula are actually serving in the test group in a research project on the health implications of genetically modified soy products and infants health outcomes.

Infant Formula of the Past
From the 1860s to the early 1960s sweetened condensed milk was the most used commercial base for infant nutrition. From the 1950s to 1970s sweetened condensed milk was gradually replaced by full-cream and half cream powered milk, and then by infant formula as we know it today (Newton, 1999). Commercial infant formula has undergone many changes since its development. The infants who consumed the initial product may not have been receiving a food that would give them all the nutrients that they needed to grow and thrive. Unfortunately, only after new research was uncovered and/or infants began showing up with deficiencies and illnesses, were there modifications made to the ingredients and supplementations added. The packaging and distribution of infant formula has seen changes throughout the years as well. Below are some to the infant formula problems of the past that have been documented:

Electrolytes
The amounts of electrolytes (sodium, chloride and potassium) that were in infant formula in the 1960s were at extremely high levels compared to the levels in human milk. This presented a greater problem when mothers would add additional formula powder instead of the recommended amounts, and the infant would be receiving even larger amounts of electrolytes. Infants who received these larger doses were at great danger of suffering from a condition known as hypertonic dehydration. After research findings were

explored, by 1976 the infant formula manufacturers reduced the levels of the electrolytes in all infant formula (Taitz & Byers, 1973).

Fatty Acids
The fatty acid composition of infant formula has undergone quite a bit of changes over the years. It has been known since the early 1960s that fatty acids are essential to the growth and development of infants. In the beginning of infant formula production, the primary ingredient use to obtain the necessary fatty acids was butterfat from cow's milk. To meet new recommendation regarding the essential fatty acid linoleic (LA), in 1976 the primary ingredient was changed from butter fat to vegetable oil. This change did not come without compromise. It was not recognized until the late 1980s that in addition to the essential fatty acid LA, that another essential fatty acid linolenic acid (LNA) was needed as a dietary source too. For these two fatty acids to operate properly the ratio between the two must be favorable. For a great many years, infant formula had an unfavorable LA to LNA ratio. The LA was high and the LNA was too low when compared to human milk (Cuthberton, 1999). It wasn't until the 1990s that the importance of LNA was fully understood. There was a modification to the LNA content in the early 1990s. From 1975 to 1992 approximately a twenty-year span, the infants receiving these formulas may not have been receiving a product with a fatty acid composition to provide them with optimal growth and development (Cuthberton, 1999).

Chloride Deficiency
In 1978-79, it was discovered that the company Syntex, who produced two soy- based infant formulas had produced a produce that was deficient in chloride (Miller, 1989). The Syntex Company was attempting to reduce the amount of sodium, however by reducing the amount of sodium, the chloride content was reduced to

dangerously low levels. It was estimated that thousands of infants were fed this formula that was deficient in chloride. As a result of this problem, the Infant Formula Act of 1980 was established. This act established the regulations for infant formula manufacturers regarding manufacturing practices, testing for nutrients and other topics related to the distribution of infant formula.

Lead
In the early 1970s infant formula was packaged in lead seamed cans. Most of the dietary lead that infants received came from the lead that was present in the cans that seeped into the formula. After the lead content was found to be extremely high, the infant formula manufacturers tried several techniques to reduce the lead content of their product. In 1978 the packaging was changed to non-soldered cans which reduced the concentration of lead in infant formula (Formon, 1987).

Taurine
Taurine is the second most abundant amino acid in human milk. There is a much lower concentration of taurine in cow's milk and soy protein contains no taurine. In the early 1970s through 1980, research began to uncover that taurine deficiency in cats had the possibility of producing eye problems and blindness, and monkeys who were fed formula without taurine supplementation showed signs of renal abnormalities (MacLean & Benson, 1989). Further research was conducted and it was determined that the taurine levels in the brain did not change in breastfed infants but did change in formula-fed infants. After much deliberation from investigators, governmental agencies and other parties, in 1984 the FDA approved the addition of taurine to be added as an ingredient to infant formula. Many European countries had been adding taurine to their infant formula since 1981. In 1987, scientific evidence was provided which

showed taurine as being essential to the normal visual devolvement of primates. Later it was also determined that taurine has an important role in fat absorption, bile acid secretion, hepatic function for both the pre-term and term infant (Chesney et al., 1998).

It took approximately ten years for the process to unfold of getting the approval to add taurine as an ingredient to infant formula. All the formula-fed infants in the United States before 1984 received a product that did not provide them with the amino acid taurine which was later determined to be essential for normal visual development and a host of other bodily functions. The research was important in uncovering the role of taurine in nutrition. However, the infants receiving human milk as their nutrition even before the research became clear, received a food that was providing them with a necessary amino acid that would later be determined to be essential to visual development and to other bodily functions. Those infants receiving infant formula during that time was not as lucky.

Infant Formula of Today
Iron
In response to the high rates of iron deficiency and iron deficiency anemia, infant formula was fortified with 10-12 mg/l of iron in the early 1970s (Iron fortification, 1999). Infant formula with low-iron is still being produced and marketed in the United States. This formula accounts for 9-30% of the elective formula sales in the United States (Iron fortification, 1999). Health care professionals continue to recommend its use, and infant formula manufacturers continue to sell and market low-iron infant formula when it has been documented that this formula could lead to iron deficiency. Iron deficiency is one of the most prevalent nutritional deficiency worldwide, and is still quite common among African Americans.

Infant formula manufacturers are reluctant, and have no sense of urgency to discontinue this product when the demand is so high and there is so much profit to be made. Some suggest that because the level of iron in human milk is a great deal lower than the amount of iron found in iron-fortified infant formula, it is justified to continue the use of low-iron infant formula. The iron level in human milk is indeed lower than that found in iron-fortified infant formula but the absorption rate is much higher.

Aluminum

Aluminum is an abundant part of the earth. Scientist are still trying to determine its actual role in the human body. Humans are exposed to aluminum in the environment and it is detectable in human bone and brain tissue. One of the primary sources of aluminum contamination is infant formula. The amount of aluminum in infant formula is extremely high in comparison to human milk. The amount that is in infant formula varies greatly depending on the infant formula manufacturer. Research has shown that the aluminum content of infant formula could be between 3 to 23 times higher than human milk (Lorenzo, Cocho, Goldart, & Fraga, 1999). The amount of aluminum in soy-based infant formula is even higher than that of cow-based infant formula. The aluminum that is found in infant formula is byproducts of the ingredients used in infant formula. Aluminum may interfere with processes in the cells of the nervous system and other tissues. Researchers have suggested that the aluminum content in infant formula could be decreased by 70% if the infant formula manufacturers would alter their processing and use low-aluminum components instead of the current aluminum products (Lorenzo et al., 1999).

Table 3 Aluminum content of human milk and infant formula

Source	Levels
Human Milk	4-65 mg/l
Cow' based infant formula	15-400mg/l
Soy based infant formula	500-2400mg/l
Premature Infant Formula	100-600mg/l

Manganese

Not much is known about infants and manganese, a trace element. It is believed that manganese is not transferred prenatally and that human milk has relatively low levels of manganese. The manganese levels between human milk, cow-based infant formula and soy- based infant formula are quite different. Manganese levels are important because of the high retention rates during infancy. Infant formulas contain significantly higher amounts of manganese than does human milk. Three to ten times more manganese is absorbed from cow-based infant formula than from human milk, and the levels found in soy-based infant formula is even higher than that of cow- based infant formula (Lonnerdale, 1989). Also, manganese absorption is enhanced considerably in iron deficient individuals (Lonnerdale, 1994). Manganese toxicity can have adverse affects on the central nervous system (Kleen, Bell & Lonnerdale, 1986). There really haven't been any studies done which shows that the high levels of manganese absorbed from soy formula causes manganese toxicity. It has been suggested that these studies are not carried out to allow the continued use of soy-based infant formula.

Table 4
Manganese levels of human milk and infant formulas (Lonnerdal, 1989)

Source	Levels
Human Milk	4-7mg/l
Cow-based infant formula	25-45mg/l
Soy based infant formula	30-180mg/l

Phytate in Soy-Based Infant Formula

Soy-based infant formula contains phytates which are plant structures not found in mammal's milk. The presence of phytates affects the absorption of several of the trace elements, in particular zinc. Researchers have been looking for ways to reduce the phytate levels in soy-based infant formula. By using a different method of processing the absorption of zinc could be increased. Research has shown that the use of low-phytate soy protein isolate instead of the currently use phytate is another way the zinc absorption level might be increased (Lonnerdale & Jayawickrama, 1999). Unfortunately for infants, reducing the phytate levels of soy-based infant formula would be costly, and whether or not this is done is determined by the infant formula manufacturers who systematically allow profits to serve as the decision makers for changes in the design of infant formula. Also, because the phytate level of soy-based infant formula is not a hot topic and receiving much attention from the public, the phytate levels may never change.

Nucleotides

Nucleotides are the building block of DNA, and are important for the development, maturation and repair of the GI. The nucleotide level that is in human milk is quite different than the levels in cow's milk or cow-based infant formula (Pickering et al., 1998). Studies have shown that nucleotides are one of the active components that help to boost the immune system of an infant. Infant formula has been supplemented with nucleotides since 1989, but the levels are not equivalent to the levels found in human milk. There are five nucleotides that are included in infant formula in the form of sodium salts (Yu, 1998). There has been interest expressed in elevating the nucleotide levels in infant formula to reach the levels of human milk.

However, there has been no approval given to increase the supplementation level (Yu, 1998).

To date there has been no reported adverse affects of the nucleotide supplementation in infant formula. Although infant formula manufacturers do add nucleotides to their products, there is an ongoing debate as to whether or not the supplementation of nucleotides to infant formula renders formula-fed infants the same results received by infants fed human milk. There has been no definite scientific evidence that supports the premise that nucleotides supplemented infant formula provides the same benefits as human milk (Yu, 1998). The claims and benefits that the infant formula manufacturers make in their marketing regarding nucleotide supplemented infant formula have never been proven. It is important to note that research is still ongoing to obtain a greater understanding of the role that nucleotides play in human milk and the human body.

Infant Formula of the Future
Technology has offered us a lot of opportunities for scientific and medical advances. The capabilities that we now have are extraordinary. As new and exciting realizations have been made regarding human milk and its role in infant nutrition, infant formula manufacturers and others have been working hard to match these realizations in their products. Below are just a few of the areas that are being explored:

Genetically Engineered Infant Formula
Research has shown us that the many human milk proteins, milk sugars and other components work together to provide the breastfed infant protection against potential body invaders. In an effort to match many of the non-nutritional benefits of human milk, the use of

genetically engineered infant formula is being considered. Genetically engineered infant formula would mean that certain components of the product would be man-made or developed in a laboratory. Several of the human milk proteins have been cloned: Alpha-lactalbumin, Lysozme, Lactoferrin and Bile Salt –Stimulated Lapase (BSSL) (Lonnerdale, 1996). Many scientist and researchers are in the process of trying to gauge the reaction of the public to the use of genetically engineered products being used in infant formula.

Formula Supplemented with DHA and AA

DHA and arachadonic (AA) are two long-chain polyunsaturated fatty acids. DHA is essential to visual and brain development and AA is necessary for growth and response to injury (INFANT, 1998). During the early post neonatal period, human milk is the only natural source of DHA (Levine, 1998). Infants born before 37 weeks gestation are at increased risk of DHA deficiencies because during the last trimester is when the transfer of DHA from the mother to the fetus takes place. The plasma concentration of full-term infants fed formula is lower than that of breastfed infants (Uauy & Andraca, 1995). This leads us to believe that the current, fatty acid composition of infant formula is not sufficient is supplying adequate levels of DHA. There are on-going debates as to whether or not infant formula in the United States should be supplemented with DHA and AA. It is currently awaiting approval from the FDA. In Japan and some European countries DHA and AA are currently being added to infant formula. The infant formula manufacturers are anxiously awaiting the announcement regarding the approval and have already made provisions. Wyeth-Ayerst (American Home Products), Novartis Nutrition SA and Mead Johnson Nutritional Group (Bristol Myers Squibb) have licensed specialty nutritional oils under the name of Formulaid, which contains DHA and AA, which could be added to their infant formula (Papanikolaw, 1998).

Although infant formula manufacturers are ready there are many pitfalls and potential dangers with the addition of DHA and AA to infant formula. Many infant formula manufacturers are looking to add fish oil as a way of supplementing DHA and AA into infant formula. The use of isolated fish oil supplementation in infant formula has been linked to retardation in growth and psychomotor development in pre-term infants (Sawatzki, Georgi & Kohn, 1994). Another avenue that is being explored as a supplementation option is the use of animal organs to provide the DHA and AA. Research has found that animal organs are contaminated with drugs, pesticides and other toxic ingredients (Sawatzki et al., 1994). In addition to the contamination of the animal organs, there are probably many other components within the content of the animal organs that may pose a problem for infant consumption. It has been suggested that the combination of fish oil and animal organs could match the DHA and AA levels found in human milk, but to date there has been no supplementation found that equals the DHA and AA levels found in human milk.

The supplementation of DHA and AA in infant formula would be based on a great deal of technology. There are potential drawbacks to the current recommendations of ways to include DHA and AA into infant formula. If it is decided that the fish oil and/or animal organs will be used for supplementation, the question would need to be asked, should the infants who are consuming these formulas be subjected to the drugs, pesticides and other toxic ingredients that was given to the animals throughout their lives? Consequently, if it is decided that these products would be used for supplementation, the average consumer would not be privy to this information and it definitely would not be placed on the infant formula label.

Low Protein Infant Formula

The exact amount of protein that should be added to infant formula is still unknown. What is known is that the current level of protein in infant formula is much higher than the levels found in human milk. Researchers have been exploring ways to reduce the protein content of infant formula. The results consistently show that when the protein content is lowered, various amino acid levels are reduced as well. In particular, lowering the protein level of infant formula leads to Trp deficiencies. This is of great importance because this amino acid is essential to brain maturity and neurobehavioral development of infants. There have been several options suggested to alleviate the problem of producing a low protein infant formula with satisfactory Trp levels. One way that has gained a great deal of support is the supplementation of infant formula with x-lactalbumin. X-lactalbumin has a 5% content of Trp. By supplementing infant formula with x-lactalbumin, the protein levels could be decreased and the Trp level would not be compromised (Rolf et al., 1999).

The level of protein in infant formula will remain at the much higher levels until a resolve can be brought forth on the issue of the Trp concentration in infant formula. While the debate goes on, human milk will continue to provide adequate and appropriate amounts of protein and Trp to meet the growth and neurobehavioral development needs of infants. Those infants not receiving human milk and receiving infant formula will have to wait until a decision is made, and if yes, hope that the benefits that are received by infants fed human milk, they too will receive by this supplementation.

Probotics

Probotics is a term used to describe actual live microbes found in food. Bifidobacteria and lactobacilli are considered to be beneficial to human health. As a result, bifidobacterium and lactobacilli have become commercially available to be added as food supplements. Currently, several brands of yogurt have added these ingredients into their products. There is on-going research that is looking at the probability of adding probotics into infant formula. One probotic that is receiving a great deal of attention is the bacteria bifidobacteria, which is considered to be the "good bacteria" and is found in higher concentration in the intestines of breastfed infants. The presence of having the larger concentration of bifidobacteria in the intestines is associated with a greater resistance to various infectious diseases, lower rates of illness and death in the breastfed infant (Bezkorovainy, 2001). The theory is that by adding this supplementation to infant formula, formula-fed infants would be receiving the same benefits from these ingredients that breastfed infants receive. The breastfed infant through the ingestion of human milk receives the benefits that scientist and others are trying to obtain through the supplementation of probotics into infant formula; decreased risk of diarrhea, decreased risk for infections, a healthy intestinal microfloral balance and a host of other benefits. It will be years or decades before this supplementation process would actually take place, and once again it is uncertain if this supplementation would offer the formula-fed infant the same benefits that breastfed infants receive.

As technology advances and the field of infant nutrition continues to evolve, serious questions are going to have to be answered. As the mystery of human milk is further uncovered, supplementation of new ingredients into infant formula will be hot topics. Supplementation of infant formula will also create a market for various businesses to increase their profits and revenue. Unfortunately for the public, infant formula manufacturers are not required to give full disclosure of the supplementation ingredients that are placed in their products. The beneficiaries of the new technology surrounding supplementation of infant formula may not be the infant consumers, but those who stand to gain as result of this new innovation.

Homemade Infant Formula

In the early 1960s about 80% of all bottle-fed infants were fed an evaporated milk formula (Cone, 1990). Evaporated milk and cow's milk was the base ingredient for various homemade recipes. In 1948, 45% of infants were receiving an evaporated milk formula and by 1978 it was less than 5 % (Cone, 1990). Since the introduction of commercial infant formula, the use of evaporated milk has been greatly reduced. There are still those who continue to utilize evaporated milk and cow's milk as a base for homemade infant formulas.

There are several reasons why the utilization of a homemade-based infant formula recipe might place an infant at risk for deficiencies and other negative nutritional side-effects (FDA, 1997):

- The iron levels of cow's milk and evaporated milk is extremely low and does not support the growth and development of a rapidly growing infant and might place them at risk for developing iron deficiency or iron deficiency anemia (Formon, 2001).

- The amount of calories that is provided in a homemade-based infant formula recipe may not provide adequate energy to support the growth and development of an infant.

- The electrolytes (sodium, potassium and chloride) levels of a homemade based infant formula recipe may be too high and place a great load on the kidney's of an infant, and on the other hand, they might be too low, which could lead to other deficiencies as well.

- The fatty acid composition may not be adequate to support the rapid development of the human brain.

Many of the ingredients that are used or have been used in homemade-based infant formulas have never been tested for use on infants. Many homemade-based infant formula recipes have been handed down from generation to generation. Some of the recipes call for the use of corn syrup or honey. The use of corn syrup and honey in infancy has been associated with the development of Clostiduim botulism, the bacteria that causes botulism. In the early 1980s laboratory studies of infant foods conducted by the FDA found botulism spores in commercially produced corn syrup (Olsen & Swerdlow, 2000). There were changes made in the production of commercial corn syrup and repeat testing by the FDA failed to detect botulism spores in the corn syrup. It has been difficult to fully determine a link between infant botulism and corn syrup. Because the information is inconclusive, many suggest that infants not be given honey or corn syrup in their first year of life. Many people are aware of the risk associated with infants consuming honey, but less are aware of the potential risk associated with corn syrup. Many health care professional, family members and friends continue to recommend the use of (Karo) corn syrup in infancy as a remedy for constipation.

Infant Formula and Safety
For infant formula to meet the nutritional needs of an infant, a complete and precise process must take place. Like any other chemical process in order for the procedure to render the desired

outcome, exact measurements are required. Infant formula is no different. The regulation of infant formula has not always been in place. In 1940, the federal government established the first set of proposed guidelines regarding the regulation of infant formula. The proposed guidelines were accepted, and in 1941 there were minimum requirements established for four vitamins and one mineral to be included in infant formula. As a result of various problems and recalls of infant formula, in 1966 the minimum requirements were expanded to seven vitamins and four minerals. This expansion never took place because nutritionist, physicians and others could not agree on the new requirements. The American Academy of Pediatrics/Committee on Nutrition was asked to review the requirements and make recommendations. In 1970, the minimum requirements were increased to seventeen vitamins and minerals and it also included protein, fat and lineoleic acid. Finally in 1980, the Infant Formula Act was passed which clarified the role of the FDA in the regulation of the manufacturing of infant formula. The Infant Formula Act also set maximum requirements for protein, fat, sodium, potassium, chloride, Vitamin D and A. In 1986 this list was expanded to include iodine and iron (Cook, 1989).

Although the federal government has placed guidelines in place for the regulation of infant formula, what you see may not be what you get. In January 1986, labeling rules went into effect. It wasn't until this time that the actual contents of infant formula was displayed on the label and preparation instructions were required (Cook, 1989). There are several factors that can and do influence the nutrient content level of infant formula. The label on the product states the minimum level that the product must have throughout its shelf life, which is 36 months. Therefore the label may not be accurate in stating the precise nutrient content. This is important and could have possible health implications on the infant who is consuming the product. There are several reasons why the label that appears on an infant formula product many not be accurate: Many of the ingredients of infant formula are added in excess to overcompensate for ingredients that are lost during the processing, many of the ingredients do not maintain a shelf life of 36 months and therefore are not available to the infant during consumption and the heating process also could affect the nutrients that are ultimately present in the final formula product.

Marketing of Infant Formula

There has been great effort exhorted by the infant formula manufacturers to cash in on all of the profits to be made by the distribution of their products. At one time, infant formula was directly marketed to physicians. In the late 1980s there was a shift. The federal government instructed the states that they should purchase all of their infant formula from one manufacturer to reduce the cost. States at that time were and continue to be the largest purchasers of infant formula for use in the WIC program. Before this shift mothers could obtain any formula that was recommended by their physician. The shift created greater competition among the infant formula manufacturers to be the sole supplier of infant formula to that particular state. The largest infant formula manufacturers all went to war. They have been in court on numerous occasions regarding unfair marketing practices; one accusing the other of making false claims about her products and other alleged marketing ploys. In the mid-1980s Nestle' the owner of the carnation brand of formula entered into the infant formula market. They joined the other infant formula manufacturers by marketing to physicians, but they also began marketing directly to the consumer. The infant formula manufacturers have been under great scrutiny in the past regarding unethical marketing practices of their products in developing countries. The infant formula industry would hire salespeople and call them "milk nurses" and send them into the hospitals dressed as nurses to teach the mothers how to mix formula and to bottle-fed. Many mothers in developing countries would be given a few free cans of infant formula and over time the mother would use the infant formula and not breastfed, and as a result her milk would dry up and she would now be dependent on the infant formula. Most of these mothers lacked the financial resources to continue to purchase infant formula and all too often the water supply was contaminated and when mixed with the formula and given to the infants, would place them at great risk for diseases and other health complications. Nestle' in particular has received a great deal of attention, regarding their unethical marketing practices in developing countries. Currently Nestle' is the world's largest distributor of infant formula. In 1977, the Infant Formula Action Council (INFACT) started a boycott against Nestle'. INFACT was instrumental in persuading Senator Edward Kennedy of the United States Senate to hold public hearings on the infant formula issue. During those hearings Senator Kennedy asked Nestle' the following questions that are still very relevant today. He asked "Can a product which requires clean water, good sanitation, adequate family income, and a literate parent to follow printed instruction be properly and safely used in an area where water is contaminated, sewage runs in the street, poverty is severe and illiteracy is high? Nestle' answered no to the above questions, but continued to practice the questionable marketing strategies. Although Senator Kennedy asked those above questions in 1977, it would do us well as a society to ask those same questions today in the 21st century. Also, unbeknown to most people the boycott against Nestle' is still on.

The World Health Organization adopted the International Code of Breastmilk Substitutes in 1981. This code was developed to set guidelines for the marketing of breast milk substitutes, promotion of infant formula, quality of infant formula, the distribution of infant formula samples and many other areas which undermine the spirit of infant health and infant nutrition. The International Code of Breastmilk Substitutes was adopted by a vote of 188 to 1 with the United States being the only country to vote against it (Kent, 1998). At that time under the then President Ronald Reagan, the United States was the home of the second, third and fourth largest infant formula manufacturers (Lerner, 1998), a group who held a great deal of influence in Washington. In subsequent years since the International Code of Breastmilk Substitutes was adopted there has been resolutions brought forth to strengthen the position of the code. Although the United States has voted to approve other resolutions, they have not taken any action against any organization found in violation of the code or done anything to assist in the implementation of the code (Kent, 1998). The infant formula manufacturers have hired high profile people to serve as their lobbyist to insure that their interest are always out front, and that applies to both developed and developing countries.

As recently as January 2001, the World Health Organization's executive board has proposed a resolution urging governments to tighten up their control on the marketing and promotion of infant formula. The resolution would address many of the issues that serve as barrier to successful breastfeeding: work policies, HIV infected mothers, electronic advertising of infant formula via computer and etc (Brown, 2001). Once again the United States greatly opposed this resolution stating that they believed that the terms were unworkable.

Again a lot work must be done to ensure that deceptive marketing and advertising regarding infant nutrition is done ethically and in the best interest of infants. Technology has now provided us with many avenues in which to reach a great many people. We need to make sure that this new technology does not create greater health burdens for us by disseminating inaccurate health information regarding infant nutrition.

Chapter 5

Long Term Benefits

The current research that is being conducted is showing breastfeeding and the use of human milk to play a significant role in the reduction of various infectious and chronic diseases, as well as other health related issues that affect both mother and baby.

The choice of infant feeding is thought to have a huge impact on the short-term and long-term health and development of an infant. Within the African American community health disparities exist for many health issues. African Americans have less favorable health outcomes and also tend to suffer the most severe health complications as a result of these health issues. Research has concluded that breastfeeding can positively impact various health related issues for both mother and infant. Breastfeeding and the use of human milk is now being considered as a primary method of prevention, and a key strategy for risk reduction of various health related issues. To name a few:

Infant

Sudden Infant Death Syndrome (SIDS)
SIDS is a disease of unknown cause affecting infants age 28 days to one year. The African American SIDS death rate is more than double the rate of white infants (National Vital Stat Report, 1999). Breastfeeding has been shown to have a protective effect against SIDS. It was found that infants who were exclusively breastfed had a

significantly lower risk of dying from SIDS compared to infants who were bottle-fed (Ford et al., 1993).

Diabetes
More than 3 million African Americans have diabetes. African-Americans experience higher rates of the three most serious complications associated with diabetes: blindness, kidney failure and amputation (Association targets, 1998). The role that breastfeeding can play as it relates to diabetes cannot be overstated. A current public health problem that has begun to show its face now among children is Type II diabetes. Type II diabetes is a chronic health problem that was commonly associated with adults, and Type I or juvenile diabetes as it is sometimes referred, is commonly associated was children and adolescents. Recently there has been an increase in the number of children that are being diagnosed with Type II diabetes. With the sedentary lifestyles of the children of today, the increased number of children who are overweight and obese, and our societies over consumption of processed and fast foods, we find that many of the chronic health problems that once affected older adults are being seen in our children and adolescents. Type II diabetes develops at twice the rate in African Americans as it does in whites (Pinkowish, MD, 2000).

Type I
There is evidence that breastfeeding can reduce the risk of developing Type I diabetes. For Type I diabetes to develop one must be a carrier of the gene and there must be something that triggers the disease. Research shows that cow's milk and cow-based infant formula may serve as a trigger for an infant who is a gene carrier of Type I diabetes (Roberts, 2000; Marincic et al., 2000).

Type II
There is also research that supports breastfeeding's effectiveness against reducing the risk of Type II diabetes. A study was conducted which concluded that infants who were breastfed exclusively for at least 2 months developed significantly lower rates of Type II diabetes (Friedman, 1998). Another study was done that concluded that a breastfed infant has significant protection against developing Type II diabetes up until the age of 40 (Hanson, 1998).

Obesity
Obesity is the most frequent nutritional disorder in children. It is considered to be one of the modifiable risks factors associated with an increased risk for developing cardiovascular disease. Research is showing that infant nutrition may play a role in determining weight management in later years. The prevalence of obesity was found to be 4.5% in infants who had never been breastfed compared to 2.8% for those who were exclusively breastfed (von Kries et al., 1999). It was also found that the longer an infant was breastfed the lower the prevalence of being overweight; 3.8% for those breastfed for 2 months, 2.3% for those breastfed for 3 to 5 months and 1.7% for those breastfed for 6-12 months (von Kries et al., 1999; Martorell, 2001).

Asthma
Asthma is the most common chronic illness of childhood, and African Americans are diagnosed with asthma at twice the rate of whites (Starling, 1998). During the last decade, it has been shown that the asthma rates increased by 42%, and the average death rate by 40%, a rate consistently higher in African Americans (Tartasky, 1999). African American children aged four and under are six times more likely to die from asthma than whites, and boys are 1.4 times more likely to die than girls (Asthma mortality, 1996). It has been

found that the introduction of milk other than breastmilk before 4 months of age is a significant risk factor for all forms of asthma before the age of six (Oddy et al., 1999).

Otitis Media
Otitis Media or ear infection as it is commonly called, is the most common cause of doctor visits for infants and adolescents. Exclusive breastfeeding for at least four months protects infants from developing otitis media for up to three years of age (Hanson, 1998).

Leukemia
It has been found that breastfeeding a child for at least six months reduces their risk of developing childhood leukemia by 30% (Elder, 2000).

Urinary Tract Infection(UTI)
Breastfed infants have a reduced risk of developing an UTI. Human milk has been shown to have a protective effect against UTI both during the breastfeeding experience and after breastfeeding has been discontinued (Pizacanem, Groziano, Mazzarella, Scarpellino & Zonna, 1992; Hellerstein, 1998).

Vaccine Response
Research is on-going which is showing that breastfed infants have stronger response to vaccinations than non-breastfed infants. Studies have found that breastfed infants have a higher antibody response to the oral polio vaccine (OPV), Haemmophilus influenza type b (Hib), and tetanus and diphtheria vaccines (Hanson, 1998).

Cognitive Development

Infants who are breastfed for 8 months or more, score higher on mean test of cognitive ability, perform better on standardized test of reading and mathematics, and scholastic ability from the age of 8 to 18 years of age (Horwood & Fergussion, 1998).

Bone Mass

The feeding of human milk also impacts the development of bone mass. A recent study was conducted which showed that infants who were breastfed for at least 3 months had higher bone mass of the femoral neck, lumbar spine and overall body compared to infants who were formula-fed (Jones, Riley & Dwyer, 2000).

Maternal Benefits

Lactational Amenorrhea (LAM)

LAM is a proven theoretically effective form of pregnancy prevention and subsequent child spacing. Mothers whom exclusively breastfeed for six months without supplementation (solids, formula and etc.) have a 98% effectiveness of preventing pregnancy (Green, 2000). During the first six months when exclusive breastfeeding is practiced, the frequent suckling of the infant causes the suppression of ovulation and menace. Unfortunately, as a common practice within the African American community, infants are routinely introduced to solids by 2-3 months or earlier (Bronner et al., 1999). Breastfeeding does continue to offer some form of protection after supplementation has begun, but it is not as effective as when no supplementation has been introduced.

Calcium Loss

Yes it is true that during breastfeeding the calcium used to produce human milk is taken at the expense of the maternal bones. This is one of the areas sited by those who discourage breastfeeding as being detrimental to the mother's body. However, they fail to offer the full story regarding breastfeeding and maternal calcium. Upon discontinuation of breastfeeding the mother's calcium levels are regained and her bone mineral density levels actually surpass the level that they were before the initiation of breastfeeding (Smolin & Grosvenor, 2000 p.445).

Gestational Diabetes

Gestational Diabetes is a temporary condition that affects women when they are pregnant. During pregnancy some women experience elevated blood sugar levels. Breastfeeding has been shown to have a positive effect on the mother's ability to stabilize her blood sugar (Benefits of, 1994). Breastfeeding uses calories and that helps the mother lose weight, which has an impact on blood sugar levels.

Weight Loss

Breastfeeding can contribute to a quicker return to one's pre-pregnancy weight. The act of milk production and breastfeeding burns 200-300 calories per day (Dermer & Montgomery 1997). This is the equivalent of riding a bicycle for an hour. So actually the breastfeeding process offers the same benefits of caloric reduction as if the mother was actually participating in a physical fitness activity.

Breast Cancer

African American women have a lower incident of developing breast cancer than white women, but their death rate is higher. African American women are also more likely to have their cancer detected at later stages and are 50% more likely than white women to get the disease before age 35 (Dignam, 2000). It has also been found that the longer a women participates in the breastfeeding process throughout her life, the lower her risk is of developing breast cancer regardless of her life stage (Dignam, 2000).

Ovarian Cancer
One of the risk factors associated with ovarian cancer is thought to be the frequency of ovulation. Ovulation cycles occur approximately every four weeks. The ovulation process requires a great deal of work. Breastfeeding is a preventive risk factor for ovarian cancer because there is a suspension of ovulation associated with exclusive breastfeeding (Seppa, 1997). This suspension allows rest periods from ovulation and it eases the wear and tear that is placed on the ovaries.

Iron Deficiency
Exclusive breastfeeding suppresses the menstrual cycle and this has a positive affect on the iron that is lost from the mother's body. Dietary iron requirements are not increased during breastfeeding for the mother. Little iron is lost in human milk, and because the menstrual cycle is suspended during exclusive breastfeeding, there is a decrease in iron loss. Iron deficiency is one of the most common nutritional deficiencies worldwide, and it affects women in their childbearing years because of the iron loss during menstruation. Iron deficiency is still a huge public health problem within the African American community.

Conclusion

The research is overwhelmingly clear that breastfeeding and the use of human milk is by far the optimal source of nutrients for an infant. Since the first commercial breast milk substitute, human milk has been the gold standard that infant formula manufacturers have been, and are still trying to duplicate. To this day they have been unsuccessful. Scientist are still trying in this new century to uncover the many mysteries of human milk. This will be extremely hard to do and virtually impossible seeing that the exact composition of human milk is unknown. Infant formula companies have designed savvy marketing campaigns, which mislead and undermine the mother's confidence in her ability to provide nutrients for her infant. Physicians and other health care professionals have done us a huge disservice by not discussing with us all the health benefits of human milk, and the possible health implications of using infant formula. Research is uncovering for us every day that infant nutrition can have long-lasting impacts on an individual's health. The programming of early nutrition and later health outcomes is one of the research areas that is receiving a great deal of attention. Many studies conducted on animals show that early nutrition is a predictor of later health outcomes. These studies have been conducted since the 1960s and there seems to be a programming mechanism from early nutrition which could resurface in later years and have an impact on an individuals overall health. These programming mechanisms have been seen in metabolism, blood pressure, diabetes, obesity, arteriosclerosis, behavior and learning (Lucas, 1998).

As our society continues to age and we are living longer, the management of infectious and chronic diseases is critical to our overall quality of life and to our global health. There is a sense of urgency within the African American community when looking at the health status of our infants. We need to shake off the stigmas, misconceptions and negative connotations that are associated with breastfeeding within the African American community. We need to look at all the ways possible to bring forth a change in the current health status of African American infants, and re-embracing breastfeeding as a standard practice could be one of the keys. This re-embracement would began to shift the control over infant feeding away from the control of the medical professionals and back to the direction of the mother and the community, a place where it historically was. We need to examine the social and health implications of our on-going relationship with infant formula, and determine if this is indeed a healthy relationship or one that is based on false and deceptive information. We need to revisit our past, and realize: Long before breastfeeding was associated with a higher socioeconomic status and maternal education, it was apart of the African American community. Long before the many benefits of breastfeeding were documented and uncovered, it was apart of the African American experience. Millions of African American infants received the many benefits of breastfeeding long before it was considered the "gold standard" of infant nutrition. Many generations have survived literally because of human milk and its many protective components. Even now in the 21st century technology has not been able to create and formulate an improvement over human milk.

The childbirth experiences that were common to the African American communities in the early 1900s and before the use of traditional medicine and hospitals mimic many of the characteristics of the some of the smaller countries of today like The Netherlands.

This country has a high rate of home deliveries, high breastfeeding rates and aftercare for mother and infants within the home (L'Hoir, 2001). The results of this kind of lifestyle are: lower infant mortality rates, lower SIDS rates and overall healthier communities. Now we find that many within the middle and upper class are now embracing this kind of childbirth experience and calling it the safest way to deliver a child. The use of home deliveries and midwives for childbirth are not typically covered by health insurance. The individuals who chose to now have home deliveries and the services of midwives, oftentimes must pay for these services themselves. At one time this was the reality for most African Americans and it proved to be extremely successful. It is ironic that back when it was being practiced within the African American community it was characterized as being unsafe and a practice for the poor, and was looked down upon by traditional medicine. But since it is now being associated with the middle and upper class, it is being characterized as being natural and the thing to do. Another point about this issue is that if African Americans wanted to re-embrace home deliveries and the use of midwives it would probably be very difficult, seeing that Medicaid and many private insurances do not cover this kind of childbirth experience (O'Mara, 1998).

The 21st century has ushered in many public health issues that are disproportionably impacting the health of African Americans. There are still huge health disparities in the: infant morality rate, life expectancy and access to health care rates, just to name a few. An African American infant born in 1980 had a life expectancy of 7 years shorter than a white infant born in a same year. By 1990, that gap had widened and was 7.3 years, and by 1996 that gap was a full 8.0 years (Garret, 2000 p. 479). In 1999, 21 percent of African Americans were uninsured and lacked health insurance. Of that number, 13.9 % were African American children under the age of 18 (U.S Census

Bureau, 1999). African American infants and children who are uninsured and lack health insurance are less likely to visit the doctor and more likely to have poorer health outcomes. African American infants and children who have private health insurance have no advantage in terms of the number of times that they have doctor check-ups over those African American children who are uninsured (Currie, 1995). Relative to other infants and children in industrialized countries, the health of the United States African American infants and children is very poor (Rosen, 1996).

As a result of the dismal health disparities seen within various ethnic groups, former President Bill Clinton in 1997 launched an initiative to "Eliminate Health Disparities." The goal was to focus on six key areas: infant mortality, diabetes, immunizations, HIV/AIDS, cancer screening and management and cardiovascular disease. Also, in December 2000, Congress passed legislation which established the National Center on Minority Health and Health Disparities as apart of the National Institute of Health (NIH) (Wagner, 2001). The Federal government through this legislation is showing that they are committed to eliminating health disparities. However when we look at many of the policies that are in place as well as the distribution of federal funds in a variety of areas, it clear that the elimination of health disparities may not be a priority issue. The action button has been pushed and now with eagerness the powers that be are saying that they are interested in "closing the gaps" of health disparities. It is unfortunate that the role that breastfeeding and the use of human milk can play as apart of working to close these gaps are rarely explored. Of the six key focus areas that have been identified, breastfeeding can play a significant role in the reduction and or decrease in the risk of developing these various health issues or complications:

✓ Infant morality, it is proven that breastfed infants are healthier infants, which increases the likelihood of living beyond their first birthday.

✓ Being breastfed decreases ones risks of developing both Type I and Type II diabetes.

✓ Breastfeeding can play a role in reducing the risk of various cancers.

✓ Breastfeeding has been shown to produce a better immune response.

✓ Breastfeeding is significant in that it has an impact on many of the modifiable risk factors for cardiovascular disease.

✓ Breastfeeding and the use of human milk can play a role in infants who are HIV positive in that it can provide antibody protection as well as helping to ward off the development of AIDS.

Promoting breastfeeding as a tool for preventive health and risk reduction of diseases is advantageous for us as a society for many reasons. Regardless of the position that the federal government, voluntary health organizations and others take on the position of breastfeeding, the African American community must take a closer look at breastfeeding for many reasons. The health implications of not being breastfed are significant for African American infants and children. The playing field is already unequal and by not receiving the benefits that human milk can provide, for many African American infants it can start a chain of health related events that will set the stage for poorer health outcomes for years to come. In addition to the health disparities seen among the various ethnic groups, it would be an injustice not to speak of the economic disparities that parallel the health disparities. In 1999, the poverty rate for African Americans was 24%, which is the lowest that it has ever been, but it is still 3 times higher than the rate for whites (Nicholas & James, 2001). One out of two African American infants/toddlers lives in poverty (Rosen, 1996). Children that live in poverty have more illnesses, including a higher incident of infection during the first year of life (Bass, 1997). Medicaid covers almost a third of African American children and reports have documented that poor children in the United States are not receiving the same quantity and quality of health care as children of other developed countries (Currie, 1995). In addition to the issue of health coverage, almost 3 times as many children lack dental insurance as lack health insurance. Children from low income and minority families have poorer oral health outcomes and fewer dental visits (Mouradian, Wehr & Crall, 2000). There are numerous examples that can be sited regarding health and economic disparities for African American infants and children.

Although federal programs have been initiated with the stated goals of eliminating health disparities, the current policies that are in place do not support eliminating health disparities. The research is overwhelmingly clear that formula-fed infants are sicker, suffer more infections, and have overall poorer health outcomes when compared to breastfed infants. The United States Department of Agriculture (USDA) is the largest purchaser of infant formula for distribution in the WIC program. The cost of purchasing infant formula for the WIC program was $567 million in 1997 (Weimer, 1999). It has been estimated that if 10 % of WIC mothers would breastfed it would save

90

the program approximately $750,000 (Weimer, 1999). Several of the health related illnesses that tend to affect formula-fed infants more frequently than breastfed infants also have huge economic implications on families, the federal government, Medicaid and private insurances. Otitis media, the most frequent reason for childhood doctor visits are estimated to cost approximately $1330 per episode (INFACT, 1999). Otitis media is also one of the leading reasons why infants and children are prescribed antibiotics during childhood. It is unfortunate that the federal government and its many programs and initiatives have not taken on the cause of breastfeeding promotion and the use of human milk as a way to reduce the risk of infant and childhood illness.

It is time that the African American community reclaims its infants and children. There are many things in this society that African Americans have no control over, but the choice as to whether or not to breastfed our children we do. The benefits far outweigh the perceived negatives. African American infants struggle on breast milk substitutes. Many infants are able to handle being fed infant formula and other breastmilk substitutes, but there are a great many who suffer many health complications as a result of being fed these products. We cannot wait until the federal government decides to initiate a breastfeeding program or to provide incentives for breastfeeding promotions. The health of our infants and subsequent community depends on our re-embracing breastfeeding within the African American community.

Bibliography

Aluminum toxicity in infants and children. (American Academy of Pediatrics Committee on Nutrition) Pediatrics 1996 97;6:413-417

American Academy of Pediatrics Changing concepts of Sudden Infant Death Syndrome: Implications for Infant sleeping environment and sleep position. Pediatrics 2000; 105(3): 650-656

Association targets diabetes in African Americans. Diabetes Forecast 1998; 5(16): 67-68

Asthma mortality in young adults and children. American Family Physicians 1996 ;54 (2):777

Bass, SM Groer MW. Relationship of breastfeeding and formula feeding practices with infant health outcomes in an urban poor population. Journal of Perinatal & Neonatal Nursing 1997;11(2):1

Beck-Sauge CM, Morse M, Stephen A. Commentary on preterm births. Public Health Reports 1996;111(2):114-115

Benefits of lactation in gestational diabetes. American Family Physician 1994; 43(3):666

Benson JD, Masor ML. Infant Formula Development: Past, Present and Future. Endocrine Regulations 1994;(28):9-16

Bertini G, Dani C, Tronchin M, Rubaltelli FF. Is Breastfeeding Really Favoring Early Neonatal Jaundice? Pediatrics 2001;107(3):e41

Bezkovorainy, A Probiotics: determinants of survival and growth in the gut. American Journal of Clinical Nutrition 2001;73(suppl):399S-405S

Black, RF. Transmission of HIV-1 in the breastfeeding process. American Dietetic Association 1996 96;(3):267-274

Blass EM. Behavioral and physiological consequences of suckling in rat and human newborns. Acta Paediatr 1994; 397:71-6

Brand, J, McVeagh, P. Human milk oligosaccharides:130 reasons to breast-feed. The British Journal of Nutrition 1999; 82(5):333-335

Breast feeding reduces morbidity. BMJ 1999;318-:1303-1304

Bronner YL, Gross SM, Caulfied LB, Kessler ME, Jensen L, Weathers J, Paige B. David M. Early introduction of solid foods among urban African-American participants in WIC. (Special Supplemental Nutritional Program for Women, Infant and Children) Journal of the American Dietetic Association 1999; 99(4): 457

Brown P. Campaigners for breastfeeding claim partial victory. BMJ 2001;322 (7280):191

Calamaro CJ. Infant Nutrition in the First Year of Life: Tradition or Science? Pediatric Nursing 2000; 26(2): 211

CDC Division of HIV/AIDS Prevention, 2000. HIV/AIDS Among African-Americans.

Chesney RW Helms RA Christensen M Budreau AM Han X Struman JA. The Role of Taurine in infant nutrition. Advances in experimental medicine and biology 1998;442:463-76

Child vaccine linked to bowel obstruction. FDA Consumers 1999 33;(6):2

Coleman MS. Undercounted and underpaid heroines: the path to equal opportunity in employment during the twentieth century. Working USA 2000;3(5):37-65

Cone TE. Infant feeding redux. Pediatrics 1990; 86(3):473

Cook DA. Nutrient levels of infant formulas: Technical considerations. Journal of Nutrition 1989; 119:1773-1778

Couce M, Fraga JM. Aluminum contents of human milk, cow's milk and infant formulas. Journal of Pediatric Gastroenterology and Nutrition 1999; 28:270-275

Coutsoudis A, Pillay KS, Elizabeth Kuhn LC, Hoosen M. Influence of infant feeding patterns on early mother-to-child transmission of HIV-1 in Durban, South Africa: A prospective cohort study. Lancet 1999 354;9177:471-476

Currie J. Medical care and children: Public insurance, private insurance, and racial differences in utilization. Journal of Human Resources 1995;30(1):135-162

Cuthbertson WF. Evolution of infant nutrition. The British Journal of Nutrition 1999;81(5):359-371

Dermer A Montgomery A. 1997 Breastfeeding: Good for Babies, Mothers and the Planet [Online] Available: http: wwwmedical reporter.health.orgg/tmr0297/breastfeeding0297.html

Devitt N. The Transition from Home to Hospital Birth in the United States, 1930-1960. Birth and The Family Journal 1977;4(2):47-58

Diabetes Forecast 1998;51(2):11

Dignam JJ. Differences in Breast Cancer Prognosis among African-American and Caucasian. Cancer 2000; 50:50

Elder N. Breastfeeding may reduce leukemia. Better Homes and Gardens 2000 July;7:204

EL-Mohandes AE, Picard MB, Simmens SJ, Keiser JF. Use of Human Milk in the intensive care nursery decreases the incidence of Nosocomial Sepsis. Journal of Perinatology 1997;17:130-134

Erickson PR, Mazhari E. Investigation of the role of human breast milk and caries development. American Academy of Pediatric Dentistry 1999; 21(2): 86-89

Erickson PR, McClintik KL, Green N, LaFleur J. Estimation of the caries-related risk associated with infant formulas. American Academy of Pediatric Dentistry 1998; 20(7):395-402

Essex, C. Phytoestrogens and soy based infant formula. British Medical Journal International 1996; 313(7056):507-508

FDA approves bST for Cows FDA (1994) Department of Health and Human Services..

FDA (1997). Department of Health and Human Services.

Fein SB. Infant formula preparation, handling and related practices in the United States. Journal of the American Dieteic Assoication 1999; 99(10):1234

Fernandez-Lorenzo JR, Cocho JA, Rey-Goldar ML, Fisher JO, Smiciklas-Wright LL, Picciand H, Frances M. Breastfeeding through the first year predicts maternal control in feeding and subsequent toddler energy intakes. Journal of American Dietetic Assoication. 2000; 100(6):641-646

Fisher JO, Brich LL, Piccian H Fances M. Breastfeeding through the first year predicts maternal control in feeding and subsequent toddler energy intakes. Journal of the American Dietetic Association 2000;6:641-646

Fleming AS, O'Day DH Kraemer GW. Neurobiology of mother-infant interactions: experience and central nervous system plasticity across development and generations. Neuroscience and Biology Reviews 1999;23:673-685

Ford RPK, Taylor BJ, Mitchell EA, Enright AS, Steward AW, Becroft DMO, Scragg R, Hassal B, Barry DMJ, Allen EM, Roberts AP. Breastfeeding and the risk of Sudden Infant Death Syndrome. International Journal of Epidemiology 1993; 22:885-890

Formon SJ. Infant Feeding in the 20th Century: Formula and Beikost. Journal of Nutrition 2001;131:409S-420S

Formon SJ. Potential Renal Solute Load: Considerations relating to complementary feedings of breastfed infants. Pediatrics 2000; 106(5):1284

Formon, SJ. Reflections on infant feeding in the 1970's and 1980's. American Journal of Clinical Nutrition 1987; 46:171-82

Freed GL, Clark SJ, Cefalo RC, Sorenson JR. Breastfeeding education of obstetrics-gynecology residents and practitioners. American Journal of Obstetrics and Gynecology 1995; 73(5):1607

Freidman N. Breast-feeding? Yes! Diabetes Forecast 1998;51 (2):11

Garrett L. (2000) Betrayal of Trust: The collapse of Global Public Health. Hyperion Publishing NY, New York

Gartner LM, Lee K. Jaundice in the breastfed infant. Clinic in Perinatology 1999; 26(2):431-445

Genetically engineered foods in your shopping cart. Consumer Union, August, 23, 1999

Gillis AM. Baby's jaundice may not be all bad. Bioscience 1993; 43;(5): 350

Golden J. From commodity to gift: gender, class and the meaning of breast milk in the twentieth century. The Historian 1996; 59:75-87

Green CM. Yes, Breastfeeding is Birth Control. Heart & Soul 2000;7(2):26

Greer FR. Symposium: Accomplishments in child nutrition during the 20th century— Feeding the premature infant in the 20th century. Journal of Nutrition 2001; 131(2):426S-430S

Gross SJ. Growth and biochemical response of preterm infants fed human milk or modified infant formula. The New England Journal of Medicine 1983; 308(5):237-242

Guerrini P. Human milk fortifiers. Acta Paediatr 1994; 402:37-39

Hanson LA. Breastfeeding provides passive and likely long lasting active immunity. Ann Allergy Asthma Immunol 1998;81:523-537.

Heine WE. The Significance of Tryptophan in Infant Nutrition. Advances in Experiemental Medicine and Biology 1999;467:705-710

Hennart PF, Brasseur DJ, Delogne-Desnoeck JB, Dramaix MM, Robyn CE. Lysozyme, lactoferrin, and secretory immonoglobulin A content of breast milk: influence duration of lactation nutrition status, prolactin status, and partiy of mother. Am Journal of Clinical Nutrition 1991;53:32-9

Hertz GS. Nutrition and Jaundice: Hold the Bottle, keep the breast. Achives of Pedicatrics & Adolscent Medicine 1999;153:1002

Hellerstein S. Urinary tract infections in children: whey they occur and how to prevent them. American Family Physician 1998 57(10):2440

Hormann E. Breast-feeding and HIV: what choices does a mother really have? Nutrition Today 1999 34;(5):189-96

Horwood LJ, Fergusson D. Breastfeeding and Later Cognitive and Academic Outcomes. Pediatrics 1998; 101(1):e9

Hurley, W.L. (2000) Human Milk and Lactation.[On-line]. Availabe:http://www.classess.aces.uiuc.edu/AnSci308/

Iron fortification of infant formulas. Pediatrics 1999;104;1:119

INFACT, Fall Newsletter 1999 PG. 2

INFACT, Fall Newsletter 1999 PG. 3

INFACT, Summer Newsletter 1998 PG. 2

Jones G, Riley M Dwyer T. Breastfeeding in early lifer and bone mass in prepubetal children: A longitudinal study. Osteoporosis International 2000;11(2):146-152

Jost R, Maire JC, Maynard F, Secretin MC. Aspects of whey protein usage in infant nutrition, a brief review. International Journal of food Science and Technology 1999;34:533-542

Katoku Y, Yamanda MY, Kuwata A Tamotsu et al. Effects of the cholesterol content of a formula on the lipid compositions of plasma lipoproteins and read blood cell membranes in early infancy. American Journal Clinical Nutrition 1996; 64(6):871-877

Kaufman M. (1999, June 16,) Free Formula linked to less breastfeeding. Chicago Sun Times

Keiser JF. Use of Human Milk in the intensive care nursery decrease the incidence of nosocomial sepsis. Journal of Perinatology 1997;17:130-4

Kent, G. 1998 Realizing Infant's Nutrition Rights.[Online]. Available: http:www2.Hawaii.edu/kent3.html

Kerling K. Soy Baby Blues. (soy milk may not be safe for infants) Earth Action Network 1999;10(6):42

Kleen CL, Bell JG, Lonnerdal B. The effect of age on manganese uptake and retention from milk and infant formula in rats. Journal of Nutrition 1986;116:395-402

Labbok MH. Health Sequelae of breastfeeding for mothers. Clinic on Perinatology 1999; 26(2):491-503

Latham, MC. 1998 Breastfeeding –A Human Rights Issue? [Online].Available: http:www2.Hawaii.edu/kent/lathan.html

Lerner S. Striking a balance as AIDS enters the formula fray. MS. 1998; 8;(5):14-21

Levine B. DHA in health and disease. risk associated with docosahexaenoic acid deficiency) Patient Care 1998; 32(2):87

Levy J, Schneider P. Newborn Jaundice. Parents Magazine 1994; 69:59-60

L'Hoir M. Dutch Interventions in Infant Sleep Practices: Pacifiers, Sleepers and Bed Sharing. National SIDS Alliance Conference 2001;April 21-23

Lo CW, Kleinman RE. Infant formula, past and future: Opportunities for improvement. American Journal of Clinical Nutrition 1996; 63(4):646S-650S.

Lonnerdal B, Hernell O. Effects of feeding ultrahigh-temprature (UHT)-treated infant formula with different protein concentrates or powdered formula as compared with breastfeeding, on plasma amino acids, hematology and trace element status. Am J Clin Nutr 1998; 68:350-6

Lonnerdal B, Jayawickrama L Lien L. Effect of reducing the phytate content and partially hydrolyzing the protein in soy formula on zinc and copper absorption and status of infant rhesus monkeys and rat pups. Am J Clin Nutr 1999; 69:490-496

Lonnerdal B. Recombinant human milk proteins— An opportunity and a challenge. Am J Clin Nutr 1996; 63(4):622S-626S

Lonnerdal B. Trace Elements Absorption in infants as a Foundation to setting upper limits for trace elements in infant formula. J Nutr 1989; 119:1983-1845

Lonnerdale, B. Nutritional aspects of soy infant formula. Acta Paediatr 1994; 402:105-8

Lorenzo-Fernandez, JR Cocho JA, Goldar LR, Couce M, Fraga JM. Aluminum content of human milk, cow's milk and infant formulas. Journal of Pediatric Gastroenterology and Nutrition 1999;28: 270-275

Lucas A, Cole TJ. Breast milk and neonal necrotising enterocolitis. The Lancet 1990; 336(8730):1519

Lucas A, Fewtrell MSM, Lucas R, Penny J. Randomized outcome trial of human milk fortification and developmental outcome in preterm infants. American Journal of Clinical Nutrition 1996 64; 2:142-151

Lucas A. Programming by early nutrition: An experiemental approach. J Nutr 1998; 128:401S-406S

Macfarlane GT, Cummings JH. Probiotics and prebiotics: can regulating intestinal bacteria benefit health? The Western Journal of Medicine 1999 171;(i3):187

MacLean WC, Benson JD. Theory into practice: The incorporation of new knowledge into infant formula. Seminars in Perinatology 1989; 13(2):104-111

Marincic PZ, McCune RW, Hendricks DG. Cow's-milk-based infant formula: Heterogeneity of bovine serum albumin content. Journal of American Dietetic Association 1999; 99:(12)

Martorell R, Stein ADS, Dirk G. Symposium: Obesity in developing countries: Biological and ecological factors— Early nutrition and later adiposity. J Nutr 2001;3:S874-S880

McCaffree J. Rickets on the rise. Journal of the American Dietetic Association 2001;101(1):16

McCarthy M. Bromocriptine not for lactation suppression. Lancet 1994; 344 (8922):602

Mennella JA. Mother's milk: a medium for early flavor

experiences Journal of Hum Lactation 1995; 11(1):39-45

Miller SA. Problems associated with the establishment of maximum nutrients limits in infant formula. Journal of Nutrition 1989;119:1764-1767

Mofenson LM. Can Perinatal HIV infection be eliminated in the United States? JAMA 1999; 282 (6):577-579

Mouradian WE, Wehr E, Crall JJ. Disparities in children's oral health and access to dental care. JAMA 2000; 284(20):2625

National Center for Health Statistics, 1998

National Vital Statistic Report, 1999, Vol. 47(19)

Newburg DS, Street JM. Bioactive materials in human milk: milk sugars sweeten the arguement for breastfeeding. Nutrition Today 1997; 32(5):191

Newburg, D. Do the binding properties of oligosaccharides in milk protect human infants from gastrointestinal bacteria? J. Nutr. 1997;127:980S-984S

Newton LH. Truth is the daughter of Time: the real story of the Nestle case. Business and Society Review 1999; 104(4):367-95

Nicholas A James S. The demographic profile of African Americans, 1970-2000. Black Collegian 2001; 3:72-79

Oddy WH, Holt PG, Sly PD Read AW. Association between breastfeeding and asthma in 6 year old children: Findings of a prospective birth cohort study. BMJ 1999;319(7213):813-819

O'Mara P. Birth Choices: A Matter of Money. Mothering. 1998; 1:74

Olsen SJ, Swerdlow DL. Risk of infant botulism from corn syrup. The Pediatric Infectious Disease Journal 2000; 19(16):584-585

Palmer B. The influence of Breastfeeding on the Development of the Oral Cavity: A commentary
 Patient Care 1998; 32(2):87

Papanikolaw J. New players enter PUFA market as products, applications emerge. Chemical Market Reporter 1998 254;(20):9

Piccianco MF, Smiciklas-Wright MF, Birch H, Mitchell LL, Murray-Kolb DC, McConahy L, Kristen L. Nutritional Guidance is needed during transition in early childhood. Pediatric 2000;106(4):109

PickeringLK, Granoff DM, Erickson JRM, Cordie ML, Schaller CT, Winship JP, Paule TR, Hilty CL, Milo D. Modulation of the immune system by human milk and infant formula containing nucleotides. Pediatrics 1998; 101(2): 242

Pisacane A, Graziano L, Mazzarella G, Scarpellino B Zona G. Breastfeeding and urinary tract infection. J Pediatr 1992;120:87-89

Preterm singleton births-United States, 1989-1996.(From the Centers for Disease Control and Prevention) JAMA 1999 281;15:1370

Quick B. Breast milk: It does a body good. Ms. 1997; 7(4):

Raji V, Elder AE, Gorenflo, DW. Iron deficiency and maternal feeding practices among high-risk urban children. Journal of Health Care for the Poor and Underserved 1998;9(4):381-394

Rendall MS. Entry or exit? A transition proability approach to explaining the high prevalence of single motherhood among black women. Demography 1999;36(3):369-76

Rolf J, Masire JC, Maynard F, Secretin MC. Aspects of whey protein usage in infant nutrition, a brief review. International Journal of Food Science and Technology 1999; 34:533-542

Rooks JP. (1997) Midwifery & Childbirth in America.

Rosen JF. Ingredients of urban pediatric health care: fourth world pediatrics. Pediatric1996; 6:898

Sawatzki G, Georgi A, Kohn G. Pitfalls in the design and manufactor of infant formulae. Acta Paediatr 1994; 402:40-5

Schanler RJ, Shulman RJ, Lau C. Feeding strategies for premature infants: Beneficial outcomes of feeding fortified human milk versus preterm formula. Pediatrics 1999;103 (6):1150-1157

Schwab MG. Mechanical Milk: An essay on the social history of infant formula. Childhood 1996; 3:479-497

Seppa N. Breast milk component assails rotavirus. Science News. 1998;153(20):317

Seppa N. Ovulation cycles linked to ovarian cancer. Science News 1997; 152(1):7

Sheikh C, Erickson PR. Evaluation of plaque changes following oral rinse with eight infant formulas.American Academy of Pediatric Dentistry 1996; 8(3): 200-203

Smolin LA Grosvenor MB (2000) Nutrition Science and Application (3rd ed.) Harcourt, Inc.

Sommerburg O, Meissner K, Nelle M, Lenbartz H, Leichsenring M. Carotenoid supply in breast-fed and formula fed neonates. Euro J Pediatr 2000;159:86-90

Soy infant formula could be harmful to infants-Groups want it pulled. Community Nutrition Institute 1999 XXIX ;46

Stehlin I. Infant formula: second best but good enough. FDA Consumer 1996; 30:17-20

Stroll BJ, Holman RC, Schuchat A. Decline in Sepsis-associated Neonatal and Infant Deaths in the United States, 1979 through 1994. Pediatrics 1998; 102(2):e18

Taitz LS, Byers HD. Higher calorie/osmolar feeding and hypertonic dehydration. Arch of Disease in Childhood 1972; 47:257

Tartasky, D. Asthma in the Inner City: A Growing Public Health Problem. Holistic Nursing Practice 1999; 14(1): 37 Temple University Press, Philadelphia

The low-birth weight infant. World Health Organization (WHO) 1990 67;17:68

Tigges BB. Infant formulas: practical answers for common questions. The Nurse Practitioner 1997; 27(8):70-80

Tinanoff N, O'Sullivan DM. Early childhood caries: overview and recent findings. American Academy of Pediatric Dentistry 1997; 19(1):1215

Tolnay, SE. The great migration and changes in the northern black family, 1940 to 1990. Social Forces 1997; 75:1213-38

Tram TH, Miller JC, McNeik Y, McVeagh P. Sialic acid content of infant saliva: comparison of breast fed with formula fed infants. Arch Dis Child 1997;77: 315-318

True insufficient milk syndrome is rare. Journal of Lactation 1998; 14(2):143

Tucker ME. Vitamin D Wards Off Rickets in Breast-Fed Infants. Family Practice News 2000; 30(24):17

U.S Census Bureau (2000) HIV and AIDS in America an epidemic with many faces.

U.S Census Bureau 1999 Health Insurance Coverage

Uauy R, Andraca ID. Human milk and breastfeeding for optimal mental development. J. Nutr 1995;125: 2278S-2280S

Udall JN, Suskind RM. Cow's milk versus formula in older infants: consequences of human nutrition. Acta Paediatr 1999; 430:61-67

von Kries R, Koletzo B, Saverwald T, von Mutius E, Barnert D, Grunert V, von Voss H. Breast feeding and obesity; cross sectional study. BMJ 1999;319:174-150

Wagner CG. Minority Health. Futurist 2001 35;(3):12-13

Wagner CL, Anderson DM. Special properties of human milk. Clinical Pediatric 1996; 35(6):283

Walker, M. Known contaminants found in infant formula. Mothering 2000: 67

Warner, G. Black infant health: Where to in the 21st century? Review of Black Political Economy 1999; 26(4):29-54

Weaver LT, Arthur HML, Bunn J, Thomas JE. Human milk IgA concentration during the first year of lactation. Arch Dis Child 1998; 78:235-239

Weber F, Woodridge MW, Baum JD. An ultrasonographic study of the organisation of sucking and swallowing by newborn infants. Developmental Medicine & Child Neurology 1986;28:19-24

Weimer, JP. Breastfeeding: health and economic issues. Food Review 1999;22(2):31

Williams AF. Human milk and the preterm baby: mothers should breastfeed. BMJ 1993; 306(6893):1628

Winberg J, Porter RH. Olfaction and human neonatal behavior: clinical implications. Acta Paediatr 1998 ;87:6-10

Wolf J. "Mercenary hireling" or " a great blessing"? Doctors' and mother's conflicted perceptions of wet nurses and the ramifications for infant feeding in Chicago 1871-1961. Journal of Social History. 1999; 33(1):97-120

Wright AL, Bauer M, Naylor A, Sutcliffe E, Clark L. Increasing breastfeeding rates to reduce infant illness at the community level. Pediatrics 1998;101(5):837

Wright AL, Schanler RJ. Symposium: Accomplishments in child nutrition during the 20th century— The resurgence of breastfeeding at the end of the second millennium. Journal of Nutrition 2001;2: 421S-425S

Yamey G. The milk of human kindness. BMJ 2001; 7277:57-58

Yasuo T, Matsushita S, Shinoda K Yoshida S. Development of perioral muscle activity during suckling in infants: a cross-sectional and follow-up study. Developmental medicine and child neurology 1998;40(5):344-8

Yip R. Iron deficiency(*). (iron deficieincy anemia) Bulletin of the World Health Organization 1998;76(2):S122

Yu V. The role of dietary nucleotides in neonatal and infant nutrition. Singapore Med J 1998; 39(4):145

Index

About the Author

Mishawn Purnell-O'Neal has been in the field of public health for over ten years. She has conducted numerous seminars and presentations on a variety of health related topics.

She holds a Masters in Public Health from Benedictine University. She also serves as Adjunct Faculty within the Health Departments of various community colleges within the Chicagoland area.

She is active on various committees and associations serving as an advocate for public health issues. She has a special interest in maternal child health issues and the elimination of health disparities.

She is also married, the mother of one and resides in Forest Park, IL.